The True Nature of Healing

A Surgeon's Soul Journey

Amy -
with gratitude for
sharing your journey with
me.   Marilyn Mitchell

Marilyn Mitchell, M.D.

The True Nature of Healing
A Surgeon's Soul Journey

ISBN: 978-1-7335332-0-1

For Jessica and Olivia
my dearest teachers

∽

Thanks for choosing me.

Contents

Acknowledgements

FIRST AND FOREMOST, I want to express my deepest gratitude to the many patients who have entrusted me with their health. The love, trust, and support you have shown me in our journeys together has taught me more than I could have learned in any school. Thank you for your great courage and willingness to heal.

Thank you to my precious circle of women friends: Laura Oppenheimer, Jeanne Hanson, Jane Hanson, Peggy Ulrich-Nims, and Dorritt Bern. Our many decades circle has been such a blessing to my growth. I can't thank you enough for your encouragement to keep following my healing path, and for celebrating with me the birth of this book. Our "perfect love and perfect trust" has been a constant source of support. A special thanks to Laura Oppenheimer for your masterful and intuitive editorial support, as well as your loving persistence in encouraging my inspiration to come forth in the world. Because you know me and my voice so well, you helped bring my message forward more clearly.

To my friend and soul sister, Kathy Ballard, you have been there for me since we were teens. Thank you for your amazing ability to see into my soul. What a gift to be known and loved so well. Your support and love have been invaluable in my growth and my healing, and your influence shines through each page of this book.

To my dear friend and nurse for nearly three decades, Marge Babcock. Thank you for being my cheerleader, my encourager, and my confidante for most of my career. We have been a perfect team, intuitive for our patients. It has been a great joy to work and share life with you.

To my friend and teaching buddy, Roberta Leenhouts, thank you for your partnership in bringing healing into a medical setting. Your healing, nursing, administration, and teaching skills were the perfect assets to begin to make that dream a reality. You have been a mentor for me by bringing such a genuine blend of inspiration and practicality to this work.

To Norah Edelstein, friend and master coach, much gratitude for your loving and brilliant way of guiding me to bring my essence into form. You have believed in me as an author, and helped me to manifest this book.

I have been blessed to have the support of a number of physician friends and colleagues: Dr. Carl Cucco, Dr. Michael Kinney, Dr. Alan Loren, Dr. Randall Kahan, Dr. Lawrence Wolin, Dr. Mary Farhi, Dr. Julian Schink. Thank you for your open-mindedness and encouragement. It is physicians like you who keep me believing that we all want what is best for our patients.

Special thanks and blessings for our healers: Janet Zachary, Laura Clark, Jill Davis, Sue Topping, Gwen Rubis, Maureen Undine. Your dedication and willingness to grow has edified all of us, and laid a foundation for the healers who come after you.

Laura Clark, dear friend, thank you for your ever peaceful and supportive presence. Your support in all aspects of our work has been invaluable. Your artistic ability has been especially helpful in designing this book. You are a light in my world.

Jane Miller, friend and guide, you have been a blessing in my life. Thank you for your expert connecting and outreach skills. You have come alongside me so many times to help me bring forward my message, with your intuitive sense of direction, and oh, yes...your fabulously delightful quick wit.

Special love and gratitude belong to Wendy Rohm. You brought my writing voice to life, and inspired me in my growth... with your ever encouraging, "keep going". Thank you for helping me see what I might be... and helping me manifest that.

Barbara Grassey, I can't thank you enough for your encouragement and practical guidance in shepherding this book into existence. You always make it such a good time when we work together!

To my wonderful family: my brother Joel...we have been spiritual buddies since you joined me in this world. You are my inspiration, guide and friend, always leading me forward. My two beautiful daughters, Jessica Fabal and Olivia Cucco: you have been my teachers since before you were born, and more recently my champions for taking my message to the next level. Thank you for loving me so well. My two little granddaughters, Zoë and Clara, are still young enough to live in perfect presence. I'm grateful for the attunement I get from them when in their presence. To my mother, who gave us the gift of believing in our perfect bodies. To my father, who explored thoughts of the vast beyond with me, loved and admired me, and still influences me from the non-physical realm.

Special love and gratitude go to my husband Eric Collins. Thank you for finding me, loving me so well, and encouraging me. Your big heart and the sparkle in your eye are inspiring and healing for me. Thank you for being there in the final stages of the journey of this book.

My love and honor go to my gifted healing teachers. Barbara Brennan, you and your masterful teachers and school launched me into the world of healing. I am truly grateful for the foundational start you gave me. Tricia Eldridge, much gratitude to you for bringing the advanced energy work into this world, and especially for the amazing impact it has had for me, my patients and the growing number of healers who are implementing this work.

I have been fortunate to have excellent yoga teachers since my college days, and I honor each one of them who guided me, as yoga has been foundational for me in experiencing the intimate connection of spirit and body. Two of my teachers deserve particular honor: Chad Satlow, you encouraged me in my healing process, always bringing me back to the heart, encouraging me to "Shine Out"; and Kathy Simonik, you always emanate such a beautiful light... your words and example have helped me to honor the light in myself.

Finally, I give my honor and gratitude to all those who have attended my workshops, lectures, and courses through the years, and my recent on-line course venture, The Access Vitality Circle attendees. You have provided me with the opportunity to learn what works in guiding people to access their true healing potential. I honor your engagement and commitment to healing. Thank you for all you have given me. It has been invaluable in leading me to understand the true nature of healing.

Introduction

ONE OF MY EARLIEST memories as a child is of playing with my two younger brothers outside (in our back yard or at the park) always under the watchful eye of our mother. As she watched us play, she would enjoy, even marvel at the perfection of our bodies, saying things like, "Isn't it wonderful how perfectly your body works! Look at what you can do! It's a miracle." As children we were encouraged to notice and value the perfection of our bodies. This extended to illness as well. We were rarely sick, but if we did get a cold or a minor injury, we felt secure that everything would clear and heal quickly. We were immune to anxiety and sleep disturbance. At the time, we had no idea how fortunate we were to take for granted that our bodies would work perfectly. This was hard wired into our beliefs and it became truth for us: we expected that our bodies would handle whatever came along and that is what has happened. It wasn't until I was a practicing physician many years later that I truly appreciated the power of this early programming. This deep trust in the body's ability to heal is what caused me to be curious beyond what I was learning in my medical training.

Early in my practice I noticed that patients' anxieties and negative beliefs could limit their bodies' capacity to heal. I saw how fear was especially potent. It could obstruct labor, delay wound healing, worsen menopause symptoms, cause cancer to be immune to treatment. On the other hand, I had two memorable patients, who six months apart, were diagnosed with breast cancer. In both cases, I witnessed their decision to embrace their diagnosis and heal all of the parts of their lives that were out of alignment. In other words, they listened to what their bodies were saying, and opened to a healing connection. Their grace and commitment were powerful to behold, and both are thriving to this day. These patients describe their experience as a turning point that resulted in them becoming more alive. In addition, I have had the honor of serving patients throughout my career who have healed themselves from serious diagnoses, several of whom came to me after they had reversed their Cancer, Multiple Sclerosis, Rheumatoid Arthritis.

Over the past 39 years as a physician, healer and intuitive I have come to understand that we all are born with an inner vital life force that is necessary for our health and well-being. Unfortunately, we live in a culture that programs us to live in our heads, so our fears, anxieties, and near constant mental narration tend to limit this vital force from naturally keeping us healthy and balanced. We wind up becoming programmed to attract disease, not to trust that the body is equipped to handle any challenge. But, given the opportunity, "it works perfectly".

Our bodies are obligated to comply with our beliefs, so buying into fear of disease can create an opening for that disease. When we have a symptom, illness or diagnosis, the nature of the affliction can be a message from the body about where we have been cut off from our vitality. When we develop an illness or disease, it is not that our body has failed us, as we generally think. Rather, we have failed our body.

In this book, I share many powerful experiences with my patients that brought me to an understanding of this vital life force and the true nature of healing. I also share my own story of how I learned to "walk my talk" when I was diagnosed with breast cancer. It is one thing to understand, and another to be able to apply the understanding. I encourage you as you travel through this book to remember that everything you read in these stories is possible for you.

Since this writing, I have continued to deepen my understanding of healing. If I were to be faced with my cancer diagnosis today, I would probably not engage in all the same medical treatment, but at the time it was perfect and I experienced a true healing.

I mention this for those who may be facing a diagnosis yourself (or someone you know): choose to do treatment that feels right for you and make it a positive experience. Don't second guess yourself. You can use any treatment as a vehicle for healing when you incorporate it into your healing journey. Your body listens to your thoughts. As long as you commit to healing, and stay out of fear, you will be on the right path. And don't try to do it alone.

Prologue

Open me
  I take my stand on the Earth
  And open Heart
  Hands
  Creative belly
  Pelvis.
  Flow through me into form.
  Make me aware of you in me
    Of Who I Am.
  Coming into my own
    Loving Power to
        Speak
        Create
  Flow through my words
    My heart
    My hands
  Loving and caressing me
    Loving and pouring forth for all.
  Your flow is unceasing—
    Overflow me.
  Abundant waves of light,
        course through me, through my ready vessel.
  My perfect body channels this Source of Love,
    loves and cherishes the flow
        as it moves through—

And then works magic in the world.
Open always
    Limitless
Yet, holding the definition of body

Nerves,
    eyes,
    voice.
    Lungs, Heartbeat.
A body defined
    Enlivened by love flow
        Limitless.
In awe
    I surrender to Love.
    Let the love overtake me.
Making me truly powerful
    And giving me
        My true Self.

There is a vitality, a life-force, an energy, a quickening that is translated through you into action and because there is only one of you in all of time, this expression is unique. And if you block it, it will never exist through any other medium and be lost- the world will not have it.

— Martha Graham in a letter to Agnes De Mille

1. Departure

MIDWAY IN MY LIFE'S journey, after three decades as a surgeon and physician, I made an unexpected discovery: I was clueless about the true nature of healing.

One Monday morning, I pulled into my usual parking space behind my suburban Chicago medical office. WomanCare is a large women's health practice that I had founded with my husband twenty-eight years earlier. Prior to that, I'd done my residency at the University of Chicago, and joined the faculty at Northwestern Medical Center, where I founded the OB/GYN division of the Near North Clinic for the underserved. Over the years, my practice had spanned traditional and integrative medicine, and in recent years had taken some surprising turns.

I parked the car, smoothed color on my lips, gathered up my keys, lunch, water bottle and stuffed them into my always overstuffed bag. It was 8:10 a.m. when I arrived at the office. Why was I always just a little late? I wanted to be early today. I should have meditated this morning.

Hurrying around the corner, I noticed the first exam room door was closed. This was a good sign. Marge was just putting my first patient in the room. I wasn't that late.

I gave a nod to Aunt Betty's porcelain cardinal on my desk next to a photo of my dear father who died almost two decades ago. As I donned my brown lab coat, I saw that there were six messages lined up across my desk. A big note taped to my phone said: "Come to triage when you get in."

It was still early, and when I got to the triage room, Paulette was the only one there. By 9:00 am, three RNs would be in this room answering phone calls for six doctors, a nurse practitioner and a nurse midwife. But it always seemed that most of the calls were for me—I had so many patients in menopause, and I encouraged them to call when they needed support.

Paulette flashed her most welcoming smile.

"Dr. Mitchell, sorry to bother you first thing, but Betty Ramero just called. She was diagnosed with breast cancer and needs to be weaned off her bio-identical hormones. She really wants to see you."

"That's ok," I said. "Get her in here in the next two days."

She looked puzzled. "You're booked for the next four weeks, not even an emergency slot."

"Just put her in wherever it makes sense—before or after my regular schedule. But not today," I said. "I'm doing a healing this afternoon, and then I'm getting a mammogram—only two years late."

Paulette's eyes grew wide. "I'm so glad you're making time for yourself and getting your mammogram."

I smiled at her and entered the corridor where Marge was sitting at the nurses' station, putting the last information into the electronic chart.

"Nurse Babcock," I teased.

"Dr. Mitchell." We laughed and then hugged. It was our routine after working together for fifteen years.

"How was your weekend?" Marge asked.

Marge always noticed when I was worn out, and periodically reminded me to value myself and my work.

"Crazy. Lots of running around preparing for Olivia's graduation party." My daughter had just graduated from high school.

"It's a busy time," she said.

"Yes, it is. So, what's happening with our first patient?"

"She's having a rough time. She has menopause symptoms, and feels like she's losing her grip. Her father was just transferred into hospice. Her son is struggling with anxiety. She's really depressed."

"Oh no, Poor thing."

"She's dying to talk to you and I don't blame her," Marge said, and hugged me again. "You have two other patients waiting. One is a procedure."

Tension ran up through my neck. *I am going to be so behind.*

My hand gripped the doorknob to Room 1. As I stepped into the exam room, I began to relax. My eyes met the gaze of my patient and a world of calm expanded to surround us. As the door shut, the frenzied, pressured world of the office was held at bay.

"Hi there, Andrea."

Before me sat a slightly overweight middle-aged woman who looked exhausted.

"Oh, Dr. Mitchell. It's so good to see you," she said. "There is so much going on. "

Andrea was visibly trembling as she spoke.

"My father's illness, and my son..."

"I'm so sorry," I said. "Tell me what's going on."

"Well, there's a lot of bleeding," Andrea said softly. "And hot flashes, and I just feel terrible. I'm not sleeping well, and I cry at the smallest thing. I have never felt like this. I feel like I'm going crazy."

"You are not going crazy. Many women feel like this as they start through menopause."

She seemed reassured at first, but then I got the sense that there was something more. I got very still, and felt my mind expand. *There is something about her husband.* Odd, I thought, but I had learned to listen to these intuitive messages, so I said,

"How is your marriage going?"

Andrea burst into tears. "Oh, Dr. Mitchell! I think my husband has been having an affair. I found some emails."

"I am so sorry. You're being hit from all sides."

I suggested a game plan. "Let's check your hormones. Today we'll draw some blood. We have to get you feeling better and then you'll have more strength to address your relationship issues."

The tension dissipated. She sighed with relief.

I gave her a hug and went back out into the hallway where the air tightened and the tension returned.

The receptionist was waiting for me. "Olivia's on the phone Should I put it through here?"

"Yes," I said and picked up the phone.

"Mom, I've been calling your cell..." She sounded frantic.

"Sorry, honey. I'm seeing patients."

"Mr. Bedal doesn't know if we have enough power to set up his band on the porch. He needs to meet you at the house. When will you be home?"

"Not till late. I have to get to my mammogram. I've rescheduled it twice. I'll find a time to meet with Mr. Bedal."

"Can you call him?"

"Is Jess up yet?" My older daughter Jessica was home from NYC for the graduation celebration. "She can help."

"No."

"You can wake her up. You'll be O.K. I've gotta keep going here."

When I hung up the phone, Marge was at my elbow.

"Ok, time for Jeannie's colpo. We're going in."

I laughed. She said it like we were going on a mission.

She needed to have a colposcopy to biopsy her cervix because her PAP smear was abnormal.

Again, when we stepped through the door, the peace descended. An athletic woman in her early 40s was standing in the middle of the room wearing a white T-shirt and the paper sheet wrapped around her waist.

She must be anxious.

I touched her arm. "Why don't you sit down so we can talk."

She sat on the exam table and I pulled up a stool.

"Your PAP showed abnormal cells," I said.

"Is it cancer?" Jeannie blurted.

"Not likely, but we're going to do a biopsy to see if it's a pre-cancer or not. I'm going to look at your cervix with a microscope and take a tissue sample from the abnormal area."

"Will it hurt?"

"There may be a pinch but most women don't feel it."

Marge eased her down on the table and helped her put her legs in the stirrups. As I began my work, Marge held her hand and chatted with her about her weekend.

I pulled the colposcope forward. Marge moved around to the other side of the procedure table to remove the drape covering the instruments, out of the view of the patient.

I put on sterile gloves, picked up a speculum and inserted it into her vagina. I moved the colposcope into place and adjusted it so the cervix came into focus.

A white area was visible on her cervix. Marge handed me the biopsy forceps, and I inserted it till it reached the abnormal area of the cervix, then squeezed down on the handle to take a small piece of tissue, removed it and handed it to Marge.

"This is from the four o'clock position," I said.

She placed it in a specimen cup.

Marge handed me the endocervical curette. I looked again at the cervix and guided the curette into the cervical canal.

"You're going to feel this more," I said.

She took a breath as I took the sample, handed it to Marge and wheeled the colposcope aside.

Using a cotton swab, I dabbed a coagulating solution on the cervix to stop the bleeding.

"You did great, Jeannie," I said. "We're all done."

I helped her sit up as Marge labeled the specimen jars.

Out in the hallway, the bustle began again.

Each time I moved into the next exam room, the peace expanded and the world fell away. The only thing that existed was this patient, this moment, and our partnering toward healing.

I'd been practicing medicine now for three decades, and it had always been this way.

As I finished with patients, one hour behind, Marge said, "Oh, I forgot to tell you, Carl wants to see you."

My husband, Carl, was the physician CEO of this medical center.

As I hurried to the front nurses station, I saw Carl standing very close to a tiny blonde, the young medical records tech. A strange feeling moved through me. *What was that? Probably nothing.*

When he saw me, he broke away and made a beeline into his office. I followed.

Carl was hyped. "Olivia called--there's a problem with the catering. I already put in a call to Gianni," he said with his typical take charge way. He's Italian, and proud of it.

"OK, good. I am late to do a healing, and she's waiting in the healing room."

"Fine, don't help," he said and turned away toward his computer.

Safe again inside the healing room, tranquility unfolded, as if I'd entered a door to another world.

The lights were low, soft music was playing, and there was a massage table in the center of the room. Here, treatments had nothing to do with speculums, colposcopies, or specimen jars.

Throughout my career, a healing force larger than myself had always made itself known when I least expected it. I'd slowly begun to tap into this force and integrate it into my practice, but I was still in the beginning stages of understanding the mysterious stuff I could no longer ignore.

Later that afternoon, I would show up for my mammogram. I'd been so busy being a healer, I'd forgotten to take care of myself. It never occurred to me that the healing force I'd applied so well to others would soon become so important in my life.

2. Vision

As I BEGAN WORKING with my last patient of the day, I remembered the first time my split world—broken into intellect and spirit, the body versus consciousness—began to come together.

It was a spring night in 1991 when I woke in darkness, silence, in a dream-like state. It was 2 am and I was on call at Holy Family Hospital. The phone on my bedside table drew my attention. It wasn't ringing, but it held my gaze. I knew that it would soon ring. *A woman is in danger with an emergency*, I thought. *An ectopic pregnancy.*

Closing my eyes, I rested peacefully.

The phone rang minutes later.

"This is Dr. Berger from the ER. I have a pregnant patient with pain and no intrauterine pregnancy. It's an ectopic. She is becoming unstable. I'm notifying the OR. We need you to come in!"

Hanging up the phone, I was startled. How had I known this?

I bolted out of bed, scrambled into clothes, located car keys and rushed to the garage to start my trip to the hospital.

During the drive, alone on the road, the deep night sky, blue-black and clear, expanded around me, unfurling a blanket of sparkling stars. The moon shone full and bright. Everything was particularly vibrant. An incredibly peaceful feeling came over me, as if the vast, pulsing universe was reaching from the night sky through my windshield, filling my car to surround me with a sense of peace and wonder. In this expansive, altered state, I heard the words, "This is not the usual ectopic." It seemed normal to hear these words at first, but I soon became startled. What would I find in the OR?

At the hospital, I rushed to the OR locker room, donned scrubs, hat and mask, and scurried to the scrub sink. As I scrubbed my hands, I looked through the window into the operating suite as the patient on the operating table was prepared for surgery—a predictable, reassuring choreography. I could see the anesthesiologist moving about, focused, checking monitors, drawing medications into syringes, injecting, checking again. The circulating nurse moved swiftly and purposefully back and forth, opening packets of drapes and instruments, careful to touch only the outside wrapping, folding it back to offer the sterile inner pack to the scrub nurse. The scrub nurse stood in her place between the operating table and her instrument table, opening the final wraps and setting up instruments in neat rows, a specific order.

I walked into the room, feeling the hushed efficiency surround me. The scrub nurse stopped, handed me a towel to dry my hands, then held out a gown. She offered gloves, one at a time, and snapped them on my hands. I stood quietly, waiting for everything to be ready. The circulating nurse rolled a small cart toward the patient, opened bottles of betadine scrub and paint, and emptied them into plastic containers.

"Hurry!" yelled the anesthesiologist.

Using sponges on a handle, she began to clean the patient's skin, dried, then painted the surgical area.

I knew I had to act fast; the patient's condition was deteriorating. Yet as I stood and waited, the energy in the room again seemed to expand with a sense of peace and stillness. *All is well.* I had not begun the surgery, but began to have a vision of a surgical field coming across my mind screen: black blood welling up, suctioning the blood away, the left ovary distorted and bleeding.

"Ready!" said the anesthesiologist.

I jumped into action, moved to the patient's side, swiftly covering her body with sterile drapes. A small rectangle of skin became my intent focus.

"Scalpel." The instrument popped into my outstretched hand. Placing scalpel to skin and pulling it firmly across, the incision opened effortlessly. Another swipe through the fatty layer, down to the taut glistening fascia layer. Spreading the fatty subcutaneous tissue aside, the full fascia was visible. One more swipe with the knife to open the fascia, then grasping with clamps for traction, the scissors were used to cut open the fascia without disturbing the muscle underneath. The midline muscles were parted by cutting the connective tissue between. And then we saw it: black blood pushing against the translucent peritoneal layer causing it to bulge between the muscles. *Just as I had seen moments before in my mind!*

"Suction." Piercing the peritoneum with the suction tip, blood began to pour over the surgical field and onto the floor. Reaching into the bloody cavity, my hand went instinctively to the left ovary, gently delivering it into view—distorted and bleeding profusely with an implanted pregnancy.

"Clamp." I clamped off the blood supply to the ovary, and then we all took a moment to breathe. Hemorrhage stopped. Out of danger. Another clamp placed across the second attachment of ovary, I cut above the clamps, and gently grasped the detached ovary to hand to the scrub nurse. Next, I tied off the pedicles with suture and released the clamps.

The tension in the air dissipated, giving way to relief and joviality. It was enjoyable to clean up after the disaster—suction, irrigate, examine the other ovary, uterus, bowels—all clean and pink and back to normal. Then with precise rhythm, suturing each layer closed—peritoneum, fascia, skin with only a pencil thin incision remaining as evidence of this surgery. Tenderly wiping the blood and betadine off of the patient's skin, I applied bandages to the incision. The patient was slowly waking up from her anesthetic sleep.

"You are waking up from surgery. Everything is fine," I whispered.

It wouldn't be till the following morning that we would have a conversation she would remember.

It was on the drive home at 5 am when I sat bolt upright and it all sunk in: "Wow, this is not how it usually happens." The entire evening replayed in my mind, and I was overcome with gratitude for the connection and guidance I had received.

Prior to this night, I would sometimes have intuitive and telepathic messages (that someone will call, or the lost keys are in the den), but this was the first time it had been so consistent and so important—it had truly guided me to save someone's life.

This was the night that got my attention. I vowed to find a way to cultivate the mysterious connection, learn about this source of guidance, and to use it in my work. I had the sense that this was only the beginning.

From then on, I would see the surgical field on my mind screen before surgery, but only if there was something unusual or challenging. That sense of expansion would come over me, a tap on the shoulder—and then a picture would come into view.

A new mysterious skill had presented itself to me. I began to quietly integrate various forms of energy healing into my practice, based on my regular encounters with things that had never been explained in medical textbooks.

But I still had just touched the surface of a very deep and inscrutable ocean. It was calling me to go on a deep and challenging journey, but I'd not yet been ready to fully answer the call.

3. Physician, heal thyself

A WEEK AFTER I had my mammogram, I was back at the Breast Center. My results had been abnormal, but I was sure it was just a glitch. I was now lying on an ultrasound table.

The distorted architecture of my own breast appeared on a screen.

Pam, the technician, ran the ultrasound probe over my breast, spreading the cold gel over a wider area.

"Ok, here it is. Wait just a second while I go get Dr. Kinney."

Alone in the room, waiting: It had to be nothing.

The door opened slightly and Dr. Kinney slipped in, followed by Pam.

It hadn't occurred to me that this could be a difficult situation for my friend Mike Kinney, the doctor. His face was easy to read, with its mix of concern and discomfort. I wanted to put him at ease.

"Hi Mike."

"Hi Marilyn. Let's have a look."

Pam again scanned the area with the cold probe, and all eyes focused on the screen.

"OK. Let's prep, inject the local and then I will biopsy and place a clip for identification."

"Oh, don't put a clip," I said. "Do you think it is really necessary?" A clip is a tiny metal marker that remains in the breast and can be detected on the mammogram for future reference.

"Well, this really looks indeterminate. Honestly, it could be benign, but we really need the biopsy to know. I don't have to put the clip."

"Thanks."

Cold betadine on my skin, then local anesthetic—multiple needle pricks, then numb. Ultrasound probe with gel crowded on my breast. Then the large bore biopsy gun pressing through the skin under the probe. Pressure, pressure—then searing pain shooting through my breast. Uggggh! Withdrawal, relief. It was done.

Dr. Kinney placed a gauze pad on the site and applied pressure. After a minute, he raised the gauze, peeked at the wound, and gently placed a gauze dressing over, securing it with tape.

"You ok?"

"Yes, fine."

"I will call you when I get the results. Probably not till Monday."

"Thanks, Mike. You have my cell phone, right?"

"Yep."

Getting into bed that night, pulling up the covers, I laid my head down and thought, *The biopsy is probably benign. Usually they are.* Turning on my side, I began to drift off.

Suddenly I jolted awake. Thoughts crowded into my head. *It could be positive.* I called on my confidence. *Well, if it is, I will just have a healing to reverse it.*

✌

Two days later, I was in the midst of my daughter's high school graduation party. The weather was glorious. Tents were set up in the back yard; the cake was in the fridge. Band members were arriving and setting up their instruments on our deck—I counted seven musicians in all—and the vocalists hadn't even arrived yet. This party was for Olivia and her friend Lauren, whose father had this incredible band. Soon, the girls came downstairs but Carl was nowhere in sight.

Guests were already streaming across our lawn toward the house.

I called to our bedroom on the intercom: "Carl? Are you there?"

"Zzzzzz..." *He's dozing!*

"Come down, Carl! Wake up! People are arriving! You are the only parent not here."

"Huhh," I heard him grumble. "In a little bit..."

"Seriously, come down and join the party."

The yard was now almost full with guests—some our dear friends, others we were meeting for the first time. And lots of high school kids. I stood in our kitchen, which now was full of women, when Carl made his appearance. As I talked with other Moms about life after the kids go to college, Carl looked dazed. I maneuvered to his side and, after reminding him of everyone's name, guided him out onto the screened porch to greet our other guests.

On the porch, we found Peggy and Nancie talking to one another. Peggy was the director of the Barrington Children's Choir, and Nancie the director of the Barrington High School choirs—both award-winning choirs. Both of our daughters had sung with them.

"Carl and I just want to let you both know how much you have meant to our family."

Carl brightened and joined in. "You are so talented. It doesn't get any better." That was more like it. He was being his charming self.

"Now it's over," he continued. "I can't believe it."

Suddenly he was crying.

Both women moved to comfort him. "You are just feeling the empty nest already," Peggy said, and we all had a group hug.

As the party progressed, and the band played, Carl dipped in and out. Sometimes in our marriage he just went missing. I had given up trying to keep track of him.

Eventually, the last guests left, and as I climbed the stairs, a fatigue settled over me. I could not wait to get to bed.

∽

Sunday morning my husband found me in the kitchen. I was making coffee when he walked in. He was agitated. He stood in the doorway staring at me.

"Marilyn, the biopsy was positive," he blurted out. "I called the pathologist on Friday and talked to Kinney. It's a grade 1. I didn't want to tell you until the party was over."

I stopped pouring the water through the coffee drip, put the pot down and turned to face him.

"You knew this whole time?" I asked, incredulous. He nodded.

"I'm sorry you had to carry that news alone," I said. "That's why you were acting so weird."

"How can you be so calm?" he asked.

"It's ok, honey. I'm not afraid. You know it's early, and I will have a healing."

His tears were now welling up.

"You have to get a PEM scan now to screen both breasts," he said.

"It's ok. Tricia will be in town. She can do my healing."

Since 1997, a while after my first experience with the vision in the OR, I'd developed my skills as an energy healer and also worked with other healers.

When Thursday arrived, I was relieved. I had been looking forward to Tricia's day for working in my office. Tricia was a master healer whom I met in 2002 at a healing conference. She had told me how she reversed an advanced breast cancer that was not responding to traditional medical therapies—with energy healing. She started a healing school to teach advanced healing and I was one of her first students. Now she was coming into our medical offices on a monthly basis to do healings for our very ill patients.

As I settled onto the table in our healing room, I began to let go. My turn to receive.

Tricia swept her hands over my head and feet to clear negative energy. I felt pulses of sparkling energy start to move up through my feet all the way through the crown of my head. I now was melting pleasantly into the table.

After a while, a new sensation arose, it was smoky and filled with a tension I didn't understand. I saw before me a shadowy structure that began to surround me. Then I fell into a deep unconscious state.

When I woke up after the healing was over, I felt drugged. I couldn't remember anything that had happened. This was very different from other healings that I'd had.

The next week I went for my PEM scan. Afterward, I was certain I'd be told the cancer was gone. But I would have to wait 24 hours to know for sure.

4. Uncertainty

UNCERTAINTY. THEY SAY THAT it's the nature of life. Security in life is an illusion, and something we're always chasing.

Throughout the ages, philosophers have grappled with uncertainty. Ancient Chinese philosopher Zhuang Zhou pondered the relationship between reality and the dream state. For him, awakening requires entering into a state of uncertainty and "not knowing". Nietzsche echoes this view of life in stating that reality is subjective, and dream is objective. And, of course, the quantum physicists have the Heisenberg Uncertainty Principle, which describes the very foundation of the physical world: the better you know the position of a particle, the less you know the momentum, and vice versa. So even on the minutely microscopic level, our entire world is built entirely on uncertainty.

Statistician Dennis Lindley sums up our plight: We are uncertain, to varying degrees, about everything in the future; much of the past is hidden. Even in the present there is a lot about which we do not have full information. Uncertainty is everywhere. We cannot escape it.

Even my marriage of 24 years, had slowly broken down. Carl and I sensed the inevitability that we would divorce. Just when we start to think we know and trust something in our lives, that knowing shifts.

In the Western world, we view uncertainty as a problem. But it is particularly Zen to think of problems—such as uncertainty and doubt—as a strength. Little questions, say the Zen masters, are as valuable as big questions. "What will I have for breakfast?" has as much merit as "What is the meaning of life?"

The "problem" of cancer, I realized, had thrown me into a meditation. It was showing me something I could not pin down; it was a koan that had created an opening, or crack, in my assumptions. Could uncertainty let the light in?

"Human understanding is limited," said Zen monk Suzuki Roshi, "and we need a way to live beyond it." To live in the world of time and space is like putting a big snake into a small can. The snake will suffer in the small can. It does not know what is going on outside of the can. Because it is in the can, it is so dark he cannot see anything, but he will struggle in the small can. That is what we are doing. The more we struggle, the greater the suffering will be."

How do we see a glimmer of something outside the cage of our habitual thoughts and fears?

I went to my bookshelves for solace.

Descartes sought to discard anything of uncertainty, and found it everywhere.

Since the 12th century, Zen masters have used koans to wrap their minds around the unconceivable. Among other things, koans encourage a view of the comic in the epic, and offer a more pleasant way to live within the vast uncertainty of life. Koans rely on surprise and imagination.

As one Zen scholar, author John Tarrant, points out, koan means "public case," and some began collecting them. But it was not such a good thing to write them down and give them permanence—their point was to let them work on the mind in an open ended way, without certainty or prescription. As one immerses oneself in a koan, it slowly changes one's reality, Tarrant notes.

A legendary story says that a Zen student longing for certainty wore paper clothing to his Zen master's lectures so he could secretly write down the koans and pass them around.

Phrases were floating into my mind as I pondered my situation.

Uncertainty opens a door to the heart.

Finding freedom in difficult and uncertain times was also the way of Trappist monk Thomas Merton. In his famous Prayer for Uncertain Times, he stated that he would stay out of fear and embrace uncertainty through the practice of trust, an essential element of faith:

> My Lord God,
> I have no idea where I am going.
> I do not see the road ahead of me.
> I cannot know for certain where it will end.
> Nor do I really know myself,
> and the fact that I think I am following your will does not
>   mean that I am actually doing so.
> But I believe that the desire to please you
> does, in fact, please you.
> And I hope I have that desire in all that I am doing.
> I hope that I will never do anything apart from that desire.
> And I know that if I do this
> you will lead me by the right road,
> though I may know nothing about it.
> Therefore, I will trust you always though
> I may seem to be lost and in the shadow of death.
> I will not fear, for you are ever with me,
> and you will never leave me to face my perils alone.

> I closed my eyes and heard:
> Certainty draws the mind
>   Into a line
>   Straight and narrow.

Takes a stand.
  Closes the door.
  Puts up a guard.
But then, not knowing, uncertainty
  Creeps in through the window
  Allows light in
  Movement, air
Breathe and open
  Expand, feel
  Trust
Dwell in potential
  Possibility
Something beyond
  Drawing to the center.
Peace.

Starbucks was a perfect place for me to wrestle with uncertainty. As I sat with my Venti Passion Tea, my cell phone rang.

"Can you talk?"

It was Michael Kinney with my test results.

I set my tea down.

"OK, Marilyn," he said. "On the scan I see activity on the right side where we biopsied, which we expected. But there is also a small area of borderline activity in the left breast, too. Nothing in the lymph nodes or anywhere else. So, we need to look at that left area again and probably do another biopsy."

I felt the ground drop out from under my feet. *What was he saying? I'm a doctor, a healer. That can't be right. I didn't hear that.*

"Can it be benign?" I asked.

"Maybe, but it is right at the border of activity—one point above the cutoff. We will review your mammogram again and ultrasound the area."

What was this? It was supposed to be gone! Not only did the tumor not regress, there was an additional focus in the other breast—something more.

The news came quickly: the second biopsy was positive. Grade one, small tumor. Not scary, but nonetheless present. Why? With all my experience as a healer helping people, why didn't my healing work for me? I didn't understand.

Things could be worse. At least it was only Grade one. Tumors are graded from one to three based on cell abnormality—with one being the least abnormal cells.

Nevertheless, I was ill. It occurred to me that I had assumed I could whisk away the cancer. How arrogant of me. Instead of approaching my condition with openness and curiosity, as I encouraged my healing patients to do, I dismissed it. As if it was like surgery, I had blithely used an Energy Healing technique, which I assumed I had mastered, to cut the cancer out. I hadn't really paid attention. Somehow, I missed a crucial element in the healing process. I thought I could gloss it over, feel nothing, and carry on as usual.

Now I realized I was just as vulnerable as anyone else. I was afraid of what I might find inside.

5. Listen to Your Heart

I WAS SCHEDULED FOR surgery the next week. After thirty years of performing thousands of surgeries, this time I was the patient. As I contemplated what was about to occur, I remembered something I had discovered many years ago: surgery is a healing relationship.

The relationship between surgeon and patient is an intimate one, although rarely acknowledged consciously. I recognized this deep connection early in my career.

As a young surgeon, I used to worry about the effect of removing organs from the body. When I was just beginning to take an interest in mind/body/energy connections, I reasoned that if blocked energy was responsible for causing conditions such as fibroids, then if I surgically removed the organ (in this case the uterus), wouldn't the blocked negative energy just find its way to another organ in the body? Was it irresponsible of me to surgically remove organs, putting women through a strenuous procedure without solving the real problem?

I continued to do surgery, and continued to be concerned, sensing that there was something more to understand here. One day when I again pondered the question of whether I was doing a disservice to my patients, a calm came over me and I asked myself, *What really happens when you do surgery?* The answer was: *The patient is better than before.* My patients are healthier than ever once they recover from surgery.

And then I knew: What essentially happens is the patient and the surgeon form a healing relationship. On the telepathic, soul level, the surgeon agrees to take the diseased tissue away and the patient agrees to release the negative energy and heal. Healing happens in all successful surgeries—in the sacred space of the OR—whether it is acknowledged or not.

But now it was my turn. The surgery was to happen in a week. Would I be able to enter into this healing relationship as the patient? I had to admit that I couldn't do it alone, and before having surgery, needed help from another healer, to be open to learn what I didn't already know. In my earlier healing with Tricia, I had approached it from a technical point of view. I hadn't let myself be truly open and vulnerable. Now she was out of the country and no longer available to me. I needed another healer.

Sometimes the extraordinary comes in an ordinary package. I immediately thought of Terry Ferrell, whom I met through Tricia. He was an ordinary guy who owned a car wash in Michigan. I know, an unlikely background for a healer. He drove a huge yellow pickup truck and was a soft-spoken, gentle man. He wore an earring and had long hair the first time I met him. I always was struck by his depth and remarkable insights.

When I contacted Terry, he said he would be honored to be my healer. That surprised and touched me deeply. Because he lived in Michigan and I lived in Chicago, all of our sessions would be long distance.

This was not a new concept. I'd first learned about distance healing at the Barbara Brennan School of Healing in Miami. As soon as I heard about it, it seemed plausible. Existing scientific disciplines supported the idea. In physics, particles and objects have been shown to affect other particles at a distance, changing their properties. When we practiced it and it worked, though, it always felt like a delightful surprise.

The plan was for Terry and I to first talk on the phone, then I would lie on my bed in Chicago while he performed the healing sessions in his healing room in Michigan.

We scheduled our first session the week before my cancer surgery.

As Terry and I talked, I outlined the details of my breast cancer, my symptoms, my life, my work, and my marriage. Terry listened deeply as I rattled off the business of my life. As our first conversation came to a close, he quietly said, "In these next weeks, be still and listen to yourself. Expand your heart and let it speak to you. Your mind is sharp and active, but you need it to be quiet long enough to listen to your heart."

His words struck me deeply:

Be still.
    Listen to your Heart.

In the week leading up to the big event, I set aside a time when I could be alone, and sank into my favorite chair where I meditate.

I closed my eyes, started breathing, and heard myself saying: *I am listening. What is this about? You have my attention now.*
My mind quieted.
I caught myself holding my breath.
Breathe, I reminded myself.
    Say yes to feeling
    Don't hold back the sadness, loneliness
    You are not alone
Open up
    Breathe in
        Breathe
Breath opens to the warm light
    Flow
Relax all the way, let go...
    Let in the warm, golden light of Love.

Rise up in me--
Pool in my pelvis
Fill my heart and flow through my limbs
Out through my throat
Into all the crevices of my head
Be with me as I process.
All is well.
Healing is possible only by connecting within.

I was engaging in self-healing. Time stopped, and the moments became a cocoon of peace, as if I was catching up with myself since the beginning of time. Sitting, I realized again that as far back as I could remember, I had known the presence of a healing force weaving through life.

Suddenly I was age nine, and as I trudged up the back stairs from the kitchen to the second floor of our house, then walked along the hallway to my room, my hand paused on the door handle. I always kept the door closed—it guarded my private space from little brothers and mother. I was not worried about my father disrupting my space, he would never intrude. I turned the handle, pushed the door open a crack, and stepped in, carefully closing the door behind me. Ahhh. How I loved my room. My eyes took in the space—my iron bed in the corner for sleep and reading. The bookshelves, overstuffed with my beloved books. The small table and chairs. And then, of course, the kitchen sink left over from when my dad used to rent out the upstairs as an apartment. My room was my safe space.

Walking slowly past the bookshelf, my fingertips brushed the spines of my books. I was looking forward to reading my new one, Nancy Drew, *The Race Against Time*. But I stopped for a moment. As I stood there, a wave surrounded me. My motions were slow and effortless. Outside this room I seemed to move differently. Here I was expansive and the outline of my body did not separate me from things. I realized in the outside world a tension and different kind of focus directed my movements.

Standing in the center of my room, certain knowledge came to me: *I have been here before. My life energy goes on. It was here before I was born and will be after I die. If it has no end, then it had no beginning.*

What an odd kid I was.

⚉

Then, another moment came to me. I was eleven years old and everyone was out of the house. In the summer, we had our family supper early, and it remained light outside for a long time. It was my job to wash the dishes while my mom put away the leftovers. My brothers Mark and Joel already had run outside to play in the backyard. Mom and Dad had just left to go next door to the neighbors' house, where they often would sit on the front porch and "visit."

I had decided to stay home, in the quiet. Walking to my bedroom door, again pausing with my hand on the doorknob, taking a deep breath, turning the handle, push, and I slipped into my own world.

I heard: *Spirit is life, and it creates the world.* I somehow knew this to be true.

That night, at bedtime, as usual, Dad stood in the hallway between our bedrooms and sang all the songs from his fraternity days, and all the old songs we loved. He always ended with "Good Night Ladies," his voice high and clear.

Lying in my bed, listening, relaxation came over me. *I can talk to Dad.* He was always interested in me and what I thought. Maybe I could tell him about how Spirit talks to me and shows me the world ...but I didn't know.

Then Dad finished his serenade.

"Good night," he said.

"Good night," we called in unison.

Sleep seeped into me. I would just keep my Spirit messages a secret for myself to enjoy.

The next afternoon, Joel was in my bedroom. We sat together on my bed playing cards. He was such a good friend. I could tell him anything. He was the only one I could trust.

"I have something to tell you that no one knows about," I said to him. I was amazed to see I could speak strongly and directly when I felt like this!

"Can you keep it a secret?" I asked.

"Yes!"

I leaned close to him and whispered.

"I sometimes feel I have lived before. And that I know some things about the world."

"Oh, cool."

"You can't tell anyone."

My heart felt like it would burst out of my chest. I could share this with my brother!

Without looking at me, he whispered, "Sometimes I can go up in the sky above my head and can see myself from above."

"How do you do that?"

"It just happens when I am alone sometimes. One time I watched you and me playing in the sandbox when we were little. I thought everybody did it, but now I don't think so."

From then on my brother and I became confidants, sharing our spiritual experiences. How had I lost touch with my own direct connection to spirit? How could that be? All this time I had been healing others, using traditional medicine and alternative approaches, but not paying much attention to myself.

I closed my eyes again and suddenly I saw a white dove. To me, it was the symbol of my father. He'd been the first person in my life to give me unconditional love. He was a birdwatcher and seemed able to communicate directly with them.

Again, I saw the dove. Dad? It had been years since I'd heard from him. Was he trying to communicate with me?

As I gazed at the bird which appeared in my meditation, I again found myself in another moment in time. It was a Sunday afternoon and I was eleven years old, riding shotgun in the station wagon beside my dad. My two younger brothers were in the back seat. Mom had decided to stay behind to have some alone time, so I got to sit in the front. Dad smiled at me and I felt my heart expand. Out the window, the sun was shining and tall trees lined the country road. We were on our way to our hike in the woods. Hiking was something Dad and I loved to do. When the car pulled into the lot at the trailhead, the boys cheered.

As we began our hike, Dad advised, "Everyone stay together. Boys, make sure you can always see us. And Mark, stay on the trail unless you ask me first. There are some fragile habitats on this trail, and some rocky cliffs."

Dad started down the trail and I moved right behind him. My feet crunched on the pine needles of the forest floor. A thrill ran through me. The trees formed a dense ceiling overhead and we found ourselves in a lush cave. The smell of pine was in the air. Lengthening my stride, I caught up with Dad and matched his pace. In his zone now, we would walk this way for the entire hike, side-by-side.

Joel and Mark lagged behind, laughing and poking each other.

"You guys can horse around, but try not to scare the birds!" Dad called back to them.

"OK, Dad!"

As we came to a clearing, I sensed Dad slowing. He saw something. Stopping, I paused, following his gaze to a tree across the clearing and spotted him: a redheaded woodpecker. Dad swept his hand behind him and waved to warn the boys to quiet down. When he had their attention, he stretched out his arm to point to the bird. All our eyes trained on this bird. We moved together and silently watched as he perched on the side of a tree, pecked in machine-gun spurts, then went perfectly still in between bouts. After a few minutes, with a flurry of wings, black, white and red, the woodpecker was suddenly off.

Slowly, the spell broke and we began walking down the path again. As we moved through the forest, Dad identified the plants and trees for us. He spotted every bird, as if he possessed a sixth sense. With my dad beside me on the path, the world expanded. My awareness of him was acute—feeling him slow his pace, my heartbeat trained to his and my gaze following his to another feathered being. There were times when our bird was barely visible, but when we looked through the binoculars, indeed it was there, just the way Dad knew it would be.

As we walked, more birds started to appear and we slowed down.

"Listen!" Dad stopped in his tracks.

A melodic song floated to us from a distance...

"It's a Meadow Lark," he whispered. Then, stepping away from us, he answered the lark with his own complex melody. Dad could sound just like a bird. There was a pause—we waited--the lark answered. The dialogue continued back and forth a few more times and then there was silence.

The nature walk faded and I found myself back in my meditation chair. I realized that these early experiences with my father gave me an access to the spirit world. How vitally important my father was to me—a lifeline. An aching in my heart opened, and suddenly another scene unfolded.

I found myself suddenly in the family room reading with my young daughters, six-year-old Jess, and Olivia, who was eighteen months old. We were waiting for Grandma and Grandpa to arrive. Since my nanny was on maternity leave, my parents were coming to spend the week with us. When I heard them come through the front door, I jumped up and went out to greet them.

Meeting Mom and Dad in the kitchen, I helped them unpack all the goodies they brought. Mom decided to put together some snacks, and I walked back into the family room. I looked up to see Dad watching my daughters as they played. I caught my breath.

Oh! The way he looked at them. I love this man! I saw and felt him emanating the sweetest, sparkling, pure love for them. It filled the room. As if in slow motion, so as not to break the spell, he reverently knelt on the floor with them. They popped up from their play to throw their little arms around him.

"Grandpa! Grandpa!"

Tears sprung to my eyes. How beautiful to witness such unconditional love. Then it dawned on me. This was how he looked at me when I was their age. This was how he loved me. This is how he loves me still. I am so blessed.

My relationship with my mother was more complicated. She was a good mother, but she often told me that I was so capable and "beyond" her that I didn't need her guidance. Like many women of her generation, she was committed to being a home-maker and often was overwhelmed and under stimulated with all the parenting and household duties. I experienced her as not available to me, and she seemed to have more attention and engagement with my brothers.

My mother's emotionality seemed like weakness to me, so I emulated what I deemed the peaceful logic of men. At an early age, I learned to retreat from my emotions into my head.

My father explored all kinds of things with me, even the nature of God. When I was sixteen, one day I found my father in the living room sitting in the overstuffed chair, reading. I knew he would be there, waiting, as he was every Sunday. I plopped down on the floor, cross-legged. He put down his US News and World Report and leaned forward.

"Marilee, what did you think about the sermon today?"

I put my head in my hands.

"Don't you think Reverend Lindquist was a bit dramatic when he asked Is God Dead?" I asked with a smile.

Dad smiled back...and we were off.

We both agreed that our bodily state affords us a limited perspective, and that God and the nature of Spirit must be more vast than we will ever be able to articulate. There is a bigger force inside all of us, alive with the most incredible energy, or really the source of all energy. That feeling I had with Dad right then was the nature of what people called God.

We continued and talked about outer space: space was infinite and so was Spirit, through which we know the Divine. If we closed our eyes and went deeply inward, that inner space was the same as outer space. We both agreed God was outside of time, impossible for us to fathom since we were so time-and-space bound.

God had to be experienced: the Spirit of vast unconditional Love.

My communion with my father revealed God.

When my eyes opened, I breathed easily. Then I remembered: I was scheduled for breast cancer surgery in a matter of days. But today Terry awaited my call.

6. The Healing Relationship

WHEN TERRY ANSWERED THE phone, I was relieved to hear his kind voice.

"How are you doing?" he asked.

We talked about the fatigue I had been having, my pending divorce, and the meditations that emerged.

"Are you ready?" he asked.

"I am very ready," I said.

I hung up the phone and went to lie on my bed. I could feel, a few moments later, when Terry began to work. A warm sensation came over me. Relief. As my body let go into the bed, I began to feel expanded so that my body limits blurred. I was aware of my bones, muscles, organs, but they seemed to have lost their rigid outlines. From my expanded perspective, they seemed to breathe and be more supple. Ahh—the rigid thoughts have let go! My organs know what to do without the restriction of thought.

Waves of energy moved through me, and lingered around my pelvis, heart, breasts, brain—almost as if continuous ripples of energy swirled around these areas. The swirling energy mellowed, but continued to move, and I felt that I was floating in a sea, my awareness somewhere above my body. Diffuse. No thoughts. Peace.

Time stopped. There was just the sea of peace. Then a sensation started from deep in my chest—a bubbling fountain of energy, the whitest light flowing like liquid. As the liquid welled up endlessly, there were small dark twig like pieces of debris that were breaking free and then dissipating in the light. Old hurts and sadnesses that had been unacknowledged and had shrouded my heart.

After some time there was a feeling of relief, like a weight had lifted from my heart. Freedom. The light energy from my heart flowed through every inch of my body and beyond to surround me. Grace. With the gateway of my heart open, my soul could infuse all of me, and connect with Spirit.

Then there was stillness—the sea of peace—for how long, I don't know.

I opened my eyes and knew the healing was finished. Slowly, I stretched and sat up cross-legged in my bed. Peace was all around me. Delight.

"Thank you for my healing," I prayed. A small shiver of reassurance ran through me.

An hour later I called Terry and told him of my experience with my heart light.

"This is important for you. Your heart has been caged in. Each time we do a healing, your heart area requires opening. In order to keep it open, you need to give it your love and attention. Nurture the connection that you felt in this healing."

In response to his words, I began to feel a surge in my chest. Light energy from my heart.

"Terry, it is the doorway to my soul. I feel it."

Silence on the line. Then, "Yes. That's it..." he said.

I knew he was feeling the energy from my heart. Ever increasing waves of energy expanding from my heart—we were connected, healer and patient. There was something about our connection that seemed to be immensely important—the connection itself, the connection to another.

I hung up the phone, feeling peaceful and radiant.

I sat down in my meditation chair, enjoying the feeling. And then it dawned on me: These healings with Terry are just as important as my other therapies. In fact, they are shifting me so I can bring more of my soul forth and truly heal. I can't do it alone with my mind at the helm. How odd that the full realization of this was coming now, given that I'd been practicing as a healer for some time.

A connected relationship between patient and healer is critical to the healing process. I had forgotten. Allowing myself to honor the healing relationship between Terry and me, I was taken back to a time when I was the healer and my patient taught me about the true nature of healing.

About five years earlier, as I walked into the office for my regular day, I noticed a difference. I'd been away for a week, studying energy healing.

Though after a week away, it always feels fresh, on this day an unusual calm surrounded me, a feeling of Grace. I smiled to myself, grateful to be in the same old workplace with a new frame of mind. I reminded myself of the wisdom of an ancient Viking Rune, "Live the ordinary life in the non-ordinary way."

In my private office, I stowed my purse and briefcase, sat down at my desk, logged in on the computer, and started to read through the charts and messages piled up during my absence. Soon, Marge appeared in the doorway, letting me know it was time to see patients. I grabbed my lab coat and walked down the hall to the first exam room.

Pausing at the door, I looked over the patient's chart. She was new to me and had been diagnosed with breast cancer. I opened the door and walked into the exam room to greet my new patient, "Hi Jeannie, I'm Dr. Mitchell."

"Hi Dr. Mitchell. I am so honored to meet you. I've been looking for someone to help me, and I found you on the internet. I know you can help me."

This woman before me was at once tense and excited, and I felt my own excitement and nervousness resonating with her. Her eyes were bright and her voice musical.

"My sister and grandmother both died of breast cancer," she explained. "So, it was probably just a matter of time before I was diagnosed. When I got the diagnosis, I just knew in my heart that I wanted to change the pattern. I believe I can beat this, and I know you can help me."

Feeling her strong intention, my heart leapt to be there for her.

I learned that she was given the option of a lumpectomy or mastectomy, followed by chemo and/or radiation depending on which surgery she chose.

"So, your doctors are taking the traditional approach and being aggressive," I said.

"Yes, but I just know there is more that can be done and that is why I am here. My grandmother and sister died despite all the usual treatments, so I think I should do something different."

I then briefed her on energy healing and how it can have a powerful effect on health and recovery. I had been doing some form of energy healing for fourteen years, and was in the midst of learning advanced techniques for cancer.

The patient continued, "I know I want to have the energy healing. I'm not sure I want to do traditional medicine."

A wave of fear passed through me. I believed in the possibilities of alternative approaches, but I doubted myself, not sure if I could handle such a challenging healing. I wondered if I should have Tricia, my teacher, do this woman's healings instead.

"There is another expert doing healings here. Perhaps you would like to see her for a session."

"No. I want you. You have the medical knowledge and the healing knowledge. I just know you are the one."

We continued talking about all the options and decided she would think it over and call me back. The truth was, I needed time to think things over myself. I was overwhelmed by self-doubt. Still, the spark of connection I felt with this patient had my attention.

A few days later, Jeannie called and decided to do "every-thing"—the full medical approach and a series of healings with me. I felt better that she would be getting all the medical treatments. I didn't want to let her down.

Jeannie's first healing was scheduled prior to her mastectomy surgery. I walked her into the healing room and gave her an idea of what she might expect as she was relaxing on the healing table, and encouraged her to just receive and enjoy the process.

With Jeannie comfortable and tucked in, I went to work. Standing at the side of the table, I grounded myself and then expanded my field in a sphere around me, connecting with healing energies in the auric field, plugging into spiritual healing like a great power source. *Let me be an instrument of peace, light, and healing,* I prayed. Then I opened Jeannie's field in a similar way, inviting her soul energy to participate in this healing.

Stretching out my arm, pointing toward her feet, I traced a circle that opened a vortex for clearing out lower vibrational and stagnant energies to be transmuted. Similarly, I opened other vortices to draw from her head and from beneath her. Feeling the room peaceful, expanded and clear, I aligned with the intention for healing: to prepare her for a smooth surgery with as little pain and trauma to the body as possible, and to bring clarity and peace to Jeannie through the entire healing process. Once these intentions were stated, I paused until I felt the shift that occurs when the intentions get anchored, or "received" by the higher levels of the field. It is a felt sense of "Yes. We are connected."

Moving my hands above's Jeannie body, I blanketed her with an energy to ensure deep rest during our session. Next, I sensed into her energy field and began to clear any obstruction or stagnation. The body is surrounded by an energy field that consists of multiple concentric layers extending out from the body. Each layer or level has a characteristic healthy vibration. When the vibration is weak or distorted, illness or distress may be present in the body or psyche.

Like chakras, auric fields have been recognized by ancient mystical and healing traditions. In humans, the auric field is a dynamic energy that extends beyond the physical body and psyche, connecting the individual to time and space, and from a holistic perspective, may be accessed in healing. Energy healing brings awareness to this dynamic energy, exponentially increasing access to the auric field. Modern science now describes and measures many of these fields, and some energy field emissions are accessed routinely in medicine.

For Jeannie at each level, I would hold the proper vibration in my field until her field was clear of any stagnation and was in resonance with the appropriate vibration.

There is an important ninth level field that has a strong influence on health and disease. It is the level that holds our unconscious beliefs, represented as grid-like structures. When I reached Jeannie's ninth level, I felt a grid that jolted me. FEAR. My hands moved to clear this grid and replace it with peace. Another jolt as I encountered FATAL. I was reminded that the well-meaning medical profession often unwittingly fuels these belief grids. My hands cleared the fatal grid.

After clearing and charging the levels of the energy field, I turned my attention to the Jeannie's chakras. The chakras are vortexes of energy that are located along the vertical axis of the body and draw in life force. They are located in areas in the body that also have major centers of circulation, innervation, endocrine glands, and meridian centers, supplying vital energy to these distribution systems.

Seven chakras were identified by the ancient Hindus as the centers of prana--life force, or vital energy. Recent healing traditions have identified more than the seven major chakras which extend beyond the body above the head, and multiple minor chakras throughout all organs and systems. I addressed each chakra in turn, clearing and opening to facilitate bringing in the vital energies that nourish the body.

The heart chakra had an especially beautiful opening. Touching into this chakra, my hands cradled the outside, feeling the cup of this vortex. *Oh, it needs love and courage.* Feeling the energies of love and courage emanating from my hands, shaping and shoring up this chakra, my right hand moved into the bowl of the chakra touching some cloudy stagnation, then grasping and scooping it out--scooping again, and again. After that, relief flowed, and her energy started to move. Holding my palm over the chakra, the love energy flowed into the chakra, filling it up. My own heart opened and a wave of poignancy moved through me. *She has not fully loved herself. This is the healing she needs.*

Once all the chakras were flowing and drawing in energy in a balanced way, I stepped away from Jeannie and formed an energetic hologram of her body in front of me. On this hologram, my hands ran energy to reinforce the structures of the circulatory system, the lymphatic system, the femurs, the thymus, the liver, and the pancreas. When it was time for the breasts, my hands moved to reinforce the structures of the chest muscles and adipose tissue, following along the arteries and veins, the lymphatics, the duct system, and finally the skin and nipples. As my hands cleared and remolded each breast, I gradually became aware of a feeling, like a message, from the cells themselves. There was a distress sensation emanating from the breasts, knowing that there was going to be a surgery. My hands responded by running a soothing energy that communicated all is well, the body is safe. After the hologram restructure was complete, it was placed into the body to integrate.

As if on a screen in front of me, cancer cells appeared. I heard the number 110, and began pulling these cells, all 110 of them, from the field. When this was complete, I placed 110 healthy cells back in the field. The number of cells pulled was only a fraction of the number of cancer cells in the body, but the message is carried to all the resonant cells.

As the healing was coming to a close, I paused and felt Jeannie's vibrancy. My own vibrancy welled up within me. My hands moved above her body, flowing a shimmering vibration through each level of the field to seal the energy work we had just completed. I moved to her feet and stood, telepathically sending the message that the healing was now turned back over to Jeannie and her Higher Self. My arms reached out to run an arc around Jeannie of a shimmering high vibrational agape love, closing the egg-shaped cocoon of her energy field.

When the healing was over, I felt pure peace. All is well. I also received a healing. What a gift to be able to tap into Spirit this way. Then I realized that when I open my heart and trust, the healing happens. As a healer, all I have to do is connect with the patient, hold the healing space and allow the energies to run through me. No reason to doubt.

The day came for her second healing—the day before her first chemotherapy. I walked to the reception area and spotted her right away—always those bright eyes. Something in me stirred. Her faith in me seemed to come gently pouring out of her eyes, touching my inspiration, making it grow, making me feel brighter too.

"Hi Jeannie"

She popped up from her chair and joined me to walk down the corridor to the healing room. Already our energy was merging, a warm tingling bubble surrounding us as we walked down the hall.

When we got into the healing room, she hopped up onto the healing table, sitting with her legs dangling over the side.

"How are you feeling?" I started.

"Remarkably well. Everything so far has been more manageable than I thought. Ever since the first healing, I have felt so peaceful, and rested. I can tell the difference in my energy. My surgery went better than the doctor expected, and I really didn't have the pain that he predicted."

"Good. So, what is your intention for the healing today?"

"Well, to strengthen my body so the chemo doesn't have as many side effects."

"OK. So, we have an intention to buffer the chemotherapy for healthy tissues while being effective with cancer cells. That is a good start. We will see what else come up." I touched her arm. "Let's get you snuggled in."

After she was settled, lying down, I moved to her side and felt my feet planted, grounded, while I opened up and expanded my field. The limits of my body felt blurred, and the energy was palpable. My heart opened. Then with resonance and intention, my attention went to expand Jeannie's field.

Again, I checked the energy field levels. Most were very clear from the previous healings. *She holds her energy well.* I paused at the ninth level--there seemed to be some entanglement. My hands were magnetized to a grid. Thick. *No, it's two grids that are entangled and need to be teased apart.* My hands and fingers moved swiftly, disentangling the lines of light. As I teased out one grid to remove it, understanding came to me. The two grids represented CANCER and CONNECTION TO FAMILY, and they had been linked together. Jeannie unconsciously believed that by having the same illness as her sister and grandmother, she was connected to her family, and if she completely healed from this, she would be disloyal and forfeit her place in her ancestry. My fingers finished teasing the tangles so that the grid of disease was freed from the grid of connection to her family. My hands held the grid of breast cancer, and using my fingers as a laser knife, cut the grid out and returned it to the light. Grasping the grid of connection to family, my hands filled it with the warm light energy that flowed freely. Jeannie would now feel her connection to her family without unconsciously needing to succumb to the family disease. A shiver ran through me. This was the first time I had encountered this phenomenon: a patient who unconsciously accepted a familial or genetic disease as a sign of a loyalty to the family. It wouldn't be the last.

Near the end of the healing, I began to work on the pending chemotherapy. My hands took each organ in turn, and gently sealed and energized them, all the while offering the telepathic message that the chemo will seek out only cancer cells and the healthy cells will be immune. A cool energy gel was pasted onto the skull, inside and out to protect hair follicles. Running through the vascular system and lymphatic system with rose light and protective liners, my hands worked automatically laying down gel to shield the body. Finally, my hands started working at the port where the chemotherapy would enter the body. Flower of life filters were placed in the vessels leading from the port to filter the chemotherapy as it goes in the body, along with the message to seek out only cancer cells, and do no harm to the healthy cells. I repeated the process, and then repeated it again. My mind began to race: *I hope this works going forward in time. It needs to work tomorrow afternoon. Is that enough time for this energy to integrate? Or have I gone on too long?* Again, I repeated the process of placing the filtering disc in the port vessels. *Maybe I can set my watch and stop whatever I am doing tomorrow at 2:00, the time of her chemo treatment, to reinforce this energy work and message.* Stressed. *How will I ever stop in the middle of my busy day?* As my hands repeated the disc insertion, I heard a voice: "Peace. I will be there." A wave of calm came over me and I sensed a presence. A tall shimmering figure was standing by Jeannie in the area where I had been working. Ohhh, relief. Tears rimmed my eyes. And I knew: *This is the Chemotherapy Angel.*

Moving to Jeannie's feet, I was ready to close the healing. With arms raised, energy flowed up and out through my fingers, beautiful flowing, arced over this patient, moved toward her head, and then connected. As the flow circulated back to me, I looked up and saw a large figure standing at her head, in shimmering long robes, emanating the most sweet, pervasive loving energy. Our energies were connected, circling, making a sphere around Jeannie. Tingling, exalted. *This is magical.* The energy of exalted, unconditional love.

Standing with the energies flowing through me and encircling me, through and around Jeannie, satisfaction abounded. My attention was drawn to an area of Jeannie's field above her, and somehow from there, I received a message: Jeannie had made a soul choice to undergo this breast cancer. She was willing to go through this illness as a teaching to others. And now she was following through on that decision. Tears sprang to my eyes. She is *my* teacher! She is giving me this opportunity to learn and believe in the healing and in myself as a healer. I also knew that her soul work would be a teaching to the medical community, her friends and family, and even her co-workers. What a blessing, and what a far cry from this cancer being a random blind-side hit.

As we talked after the healing, I told her the message I received, and how grateful I was for this opportunity and for her trust in me. She looked at me shyly and smiled, "I felt that. I know I am helping others, and it makes all the difference. During the healing, I also heard the word 'teacher'".

Five days after her first chemotherapy session, Jeannie called to say she was experiencing constipation. We asked her to come to the office, and Marge put her in our extra exam room, so I could run in between my scheduled patients. She reported that she had been constipated ever since the chemo treatment, but "otherwise felt fine". She lay down on the exam table. I placed my hand over her abdomen, taking a moment to breathe and expand my field. I began to feel rose light enter my body and pulse down through my arm and out through my hand. Placing my hand over the abdomen in the right lower quadrant, the rose light was directed at the ileocecal valve (the juncture of the small intestine and colon), and then as my hand followed the path of the bowel, the light plowed through the ascending colon, across the transverse colon, and along the left descending colon to the rectum. I told Jeannie to rest a bit before she left, but in five minutes, she scurried out of the room to the bathroom—constipation cured! This became a regular routine with the chemo, so that Jeannie would plan to come in for a "treatment" two to three days after her chemo.

Two weeks into her chemotherapy treatment, Jeannie called me to say that she was starting to have some hair fall out. When I hung up from the call, I stood in my office, expanded my field and "felt" her scalp in a hologram. My fingers went to work, restructuring the hair follicles, and pasting rose gel along her scalp and eye lashes. She called me back in two days to give me the feedback that when she had hung up the phone from me the first time, she immediately felt tingling in her scalp and eyebrows. "I could feel you working on me." Her hair stopped falling out.

Later, Jeannie told me that she felt the presence of the Chemotherapy Angel with her each time she went for the treatments. She knew that the staff could feel the angel's presence too.

Tears came to my eyes, and I felt my heart open as I remembered the beautiful healing relationship I shared with Jeannie. She had wholeheartedly put her trust in me. That is what I needed to do with Terry--let go of the doubts and fears of my mind, and connect in a healing relationship with my heart.

Jeannie's healing journey showed me that there is always a deeper meaning to illness. In her case, her soul had chosen to change the inherited pattern by recovering from this familial disease while still belonging to the family. Her healing journey also gave her an opportunity to be a teacher, by the grace with which she was moving through cancer recovery to health. It occurred to me that when we go to the soul for meaning and purpose in illness, it is always profound. Often, our mind's first impulse is to blame, either ourselves or our emotional or physical environment. But soul meaning is deeper than that. Healing is always an invitation to connect us with more of our soul essence. It doesn't always mean that the illness will regress or the patient will not die, although it usually changes the course of disease dramatically. The fearful mind wants to eradicate the illness, find something it can control; the soul brings peace and acceptance for whatever life brings.

While the mind pushes to solve a problem, soul offers freedom from the problem.

I vowed to embrace my own healing, rather than remove myself as a spectator.

This was my opportunity to get out of my head and open my heart to my soul's path.

The night before my surgery I again spoke with Terry. He wanted to talk with me in preparation for my healing the next day while I was in the operating room.

"Can you tell me anything about the procedure so I can know what to look for?"

I proceeded to tell him what the OR looked like, the routines for positioning and prepping a patient, the anesthesia procedures, and then went through the typical steps of the surgery as far as I knew them. I explained that the doctor would remove the tumors and sample a few lymph nodes on both sides.

He wanted to know the precise time the surgery would begin.

"1:00 p.m.," I told him.

7. Surgery

MY FRIEND KATHY AND I left my house together the morning of my surgery. She'd driven to Chicago from Indianapolis, and my surgery was taking place early afternoon.

As we settled into the car, I felt my body relaxing into the seat. She knew me so well. I'd known her since 5th grade, when our family moved to Indianapolis from Marion, Indiana. Kathy was a year behind me, but we were both in the group of "walkers," kids who lived close enough to walk to school. Kathy practically became part of our family and adopted my mom and dad as her second set of parents. As a kid, she ate meals at our house, slept over, and also became friends with my brother Joel. As teenagers, we spent all our time together, except when I went to work or had a date. Kathy was a poet, an intuitive and deeply loving person, and my whole being felt seen and known by her. She helped me develop a deeper source, softening my mind-driven approach to life. Everything golden between us remained.

The surgery required that I get to the hospital in the morning to be prepared. My daughters would join us later.

"Where's Carl?" Kathy asked.

"Already at the hospital, making rounds," I said. "He will catch up with me later. It's better that way. He would be too nervous and distracted. It would just make me feel alone."

"Don't worry about anything. This is about you and I am here with you."

At the hospital, we parked in the outpatient parking lot. Funny not to be in the doctors' lot. Walking up to Patient Registration, a wave of sadness ran through me. Somehow, I believed being a doctor would protect me from having to walk through these doors and from getting ill. Difficult to admit.

After filling out reams of paper work, we waited in the main lobby.

After a time, a smiling woman appeared in the lobby holding a stack of booklets and papers, and wearing a white lab coat, a hospital name badge around her neck.

"Dr. Mitchell?"

"Yes."

"I am your Patient Navigator for today. You can come with me to change into your gown."

Looking at Kathy, she then said, "Would you like to come too?"

We both nodded and went together to a dressing room. As we entered, I felt odd. Vulnerable. Then it dawned on me: I had never been in the patient's dressing room.

Opening the locker, I saw two folded patient gowns and a plastic packet stacked on the shelf. I removed my clothes and placed them in the locker, then unfolded the first gown and put my arms in. Kathy tied it in the back. The other gown was meant to act as a robe, so I pulled my arms through the other way. The plastic packet contained blue slipper socks. I sat on the bench, pulled on the socks, and stood up.

Ok, not my best look. I looked at Kathy, and without saying a word, we burst out laughing. I slammed the locker door and we walked out to the hallway where I began the morning journey.

I traveled by wheelchair, pushed by the Patient Navigator. Kathy walked alongside as we made our way to the special radiology section. When we got to the doorway of the mammogram room, we parked the wheelchair.

Kathy leaned down to kiss my cheek. "Love you," she whispered.

The door opened and a technician stood in the doorway.

"Dr. Mitchell," she said.

"Yes." I stood up from the wheelchair and walked into the darkened room.

The set up was different. There was an upright type of chair in front of the mammogram machine. I took a seat on the chair, pulled down my gown, and proceeded to have a series of mammograms. After approximately six films on the right, the technician moved to the left.

During the last shots on the left, the door opened and the radiologist walked in. He had been viewing the digital images in another room as they were recorded by the machine.

"Hello, Doctor!" he smiled broadly.

"Hi," I answered. So awkward, trying to put all my doctor colleagues at ease. I didn't predict any of this.

He remained in the room until we finished, instructing the technician how to subtly move the machines to see more of the area he was trying to capture.

"Where's Carl?" he asked.

"He's here, doing rounds and surgery. He will join me in pre-op."

When we finished, the tech moved the arm of the mammogram machine away.

"Okay," the radiologist said. "Let me review all these and I will see you in the room across the hall."

I realized then I had no idea how the whole process went. It had never been on my radar except in the most superficial way—the pre-op steps for my patients. All I knew was the radiologist had to locate the tumors on the mammogram and place wires into the middle of each tumor. These would guide the surgeon when he performed the surgery that afternoon.

The Patient Navigator walked me across the hall into a larger room. The lights were bright, and there was a long patient table across one wall, hung about shoulder height, it seemed. There was also a mammogram machine, and counters with jars, vials, and packets of wrapped instruments. A mayo stand (for instruments during a procedure) was placed off center on a table in the middle of the room. This was the room where the guide wires would be placed in each of my breast tumors as markers for my surgeon

A technician stood waiting for me, and helped me climb the stepstool onto the high floating table. She explained how I needed to be positioned, lying prone with my breast through the hole in the table. Once I was in position, the radiologist would come to place the wires using the mammograms for guidance. The technician now stood on the step stool and helped me take my right arm out of the gown sleeve, then pulled the gown down to expose my right breast. I was cold. My legs dangled over the curved sides of the hard plastic patient table.

How was I supposed to maneuver into position? Pushing back into the center dip of the table, I bent my knees and attempted to pull my legs underneath me. After several tries, I folded my legs beneath me. What now? Perhaps hands and knees. Turning over and placing my hands, I pulled my legs around so I was on hands and knees. But I was facing the wrong way! How did my older patients do this? This was ridiculous. I was adept at yoga! Slowly I shimmied around on the cold, unyielding plastic, and faced the right way on the table, scooching forward on hands and knees, I reached the top of the table and lay down positioning my breast in the hole designated for that. The table was so hard that it cut into my breastbone. There was no place for my head. I shifted around trying to get comfortable, but this was it. There was no other way to be on this table. Ugh. Pain continued in my breastbone.

The technician announced that the radiologist would be right in. OK, I could do this for a few minutes. Breathe.

Five minutes passed. Pain. Pressure in my ribcage. Ten minutes. This was crazy. I couldn't believe they made patients go through this. The pain didn't stop.

Thirty-five minutes later, the radiologist arrived and took a seat by my head.

"Ok, we are just getting the mammogram in position," he said. I wonder if he had any idea I waited so long and it hurt so much?

"So, you don't have a clip here?"

Back at my first biopsy I talked the doctor out of leaving a marker clip at the site, making it more difficult to locate now. I should have just let him do his normal routine.

"No," I answered.

After what seemed like forever, he began the procedure. The mammogram squeezed, prodded my breast, then a needle prick with local anesthesia. Stinging. Then searing pain as the wire threaded through my breast into the center of the tumor. Though maybe only twenty-five or thirty minutes, with my head face down, and no familiarity with the steps, the procedure seemed endless.

Finally, we were finished. Then the radiologist noticed something on the medical report. "Oh, are we placing a second one? Two tumors?" he asked.

The technician acknowledged this.

"OK," the radiologist said to me. "You can move now so we can do the left breast."

My arms were stiff from so long in one position. I placed my hands push-up style, and shifted my left breast into position through the small hole. A warm hand cradled my back. The technician. Tears formed in my eyes. The pressure was released from my breastbone, but it was still tender. Settling in, there was a new pressure area. This was barbaric. Thankfully, the left wire took just a few minutes.

"All done, "the radiologist called cheerily over his shoulder as he walked out the door.

I unfolded myself from the table, and rubbed my arms and chest. Climbing down on the stepstool and hobbling out to the hall, I collapsed into the wheelchair. Kathy and the Patient Navigator joined me again, and we made our way through a long hallway to the nuclear medicine department.

Kathy was allowed to accompany me to the doorway of the nuclear medicine room. She leaned down to kiss my cheek.

The Navigator steadied the wheelchair while I stood and walked into the room. "I will wait for you here," she said.

The lights were dim, making it difficult to see anything but large shadows. The technician guided me to a chair. On the counter next to the chair were a syringe and a vial with the radioactive danger symbol on it. The technician put on gloves and gingerly drew the liquid in the vial into a syringe. Cool alcohol was swabbed on my upper arm. The technician, inserted the needle, piercing just below the skin and injected the radioactive dye, then removed the needle and massaged the site with two gloved fingers.

There was a waiting period now as the radioactive dye found its way to my lymph nodes. Images were to be taken of my lymph nodes. The doctor would be looking at the film to see the location of my lymph nodes, and later in surgery would evaluate the level of radioactivity in the nodes to determine which ones he would sample for cancer cells. After a while the technician took the X-ray and I was back in the wheelchair on my way to the waiting area.

When I returned, I saw that my mom and my two daughters had joined Kathy. As my wheelchair came closer, I felt their tension. Something had happened.

"Well, Carl sent us to the wrong place. Where is he?" Mom started in.

"Grandma, it's fine, "Olivia piped in sternly.

Jess turned to me. "Dad gave us directions to the parking lot near where the surgery is going to be. That's where our car is parked now. Then we found out you were over here."

My mother was in a state. "It was a terribly long walk! And Carl was nowhere in sight when we got there."

"Grandma, he never said he was going to meet us!" Olivia said.

"Well, I'm glad you found me. Your car will be handy at the end of the day," I said.

Now it was just a matter of waiting. I breathed calmly and it started to shift the mood, allowing all the ruffled feathers to settle. After about thirty minutes, my Patient Navigator appeared again and pushed my wheelchair, leading our entourage through the winding hallways to the pre-op holding area.

When we arrived, the Patient Navigator hugged me good-bye and escorted my group to the waiting area. The nurses whisked me into a cubicle and closed the curtain. After a few more questions and taking all my vital signs, they helped me onto a gurney, started my IV, and I was ready to wait again.

Suddenly Carl burst in through the curtain, and squeezed my hand. Before we could say anything, the curtain opened again and in filed my family: Mom, Jess, Olivia, and Kathy. A regular crowd! A party! As we laughed and talked, the curtain opened again and it was my doctor, Mike.

"What a gathering!" he said, clearly surprised.

He then explained the procedure, and showed us the films of the lymph nodes. He assured us he would be right out to see my family afterward.

When the nurse whisked the curtains open, I saw the OR tech was ready to transport me. It was time to say goodbye. I looked into the many wide eyes staring at me. They were afraid. It surprised me. I was not afraid.

"It's going to be fine. Don't worry, "I whispered to my daughters as they kissed me.

Clunk! The brake was released from the gurney and I was in motion. Winding through the pre-op area feet first, we passed other cubicles with closed curtains and came to a set of double doors marked "No Admittance." Automatically the doors opened and I was pushed through. A second set of doors said, "Only surgical attire beyond this point." The technician helped me put on a surgical hat to cover my hair. Behind these doors was the surgical desk.

As we approached the desk, the surgical head nurse looked up and said, "Hi Dr. Mitchell." She then turned to the technician pushing me. "Room 7."

After winding through the hallway, we came to my OR, the place where I had operated on patients many times. Strange to be entering this room on a gurney. We bumped the doors on the way into the room, and I caught a glimpse of the scrub sink.

The scrub nurse turned around from aligning her instruments.

"Oh, Dr. Mitchell, I am so sorry you are here. I am honored to take care of you."

Unexpected tears sprang to my eyes. *But I am going to be fine.*

The circulating nurse scurried over to help maneuver the gurney around and, clunk, the brake was set again. She took my arm and helped guide me as I planted my feet and shimmied over to the narrow operating table.

"You are going to do fine," she whispered in my ear.

"Hi Marilyn," my anesthesiologist smiled as he peered into my face from above. His features started to look strange upside down, so I closed my eyes.

A blanket was placed over me, and then a safety belt placed across my legs. My arms were strapped to the arm rests, stretched out from my sides. Finally, a plastic "blanket" inflated with warm air was placed across my shoulders. It felt comforting.

The anesthesiologist rummaged around under the blanket to find the IV access, then said, "OK, you are going to go to sleep now."

I closed my eyes and breathed in. Oooo-- a stinging as the anesthetic moved into my arm. Tingling sensation in my head.

I opened my eyes for a moment and looked at the clock on the wall. It was 1:45 p.m.

Then everything went blank.

8. Journey to the other world

TIME NO LONGER HAD sharp edges. I had given up control. The OR is a portal between the worlds, and I was traveling to the vast light of the soul.

Anesthesia, be my elixir
    Quiet my mind
    Open the gates
Take me to the other world
    So I can greet my soul again.
When this journey is complete
    May I awaken with a healing, a vision.
Powerful spirit wisdom
Floats in the place of no thoughts...

I have encountered soul before: giving birth to my daughter. Back then, in the birthing room, lights low, the nurse moved around the room fussing with my IV, the monitor, adjusting the bed. I'm there once more. In the corner was the baby's bed, ready and waiting. Pitocin dripped through the IV, increasing the intensity of the contractions. Tightening, bearing down. Breathing was enough. The sound of the baby's heartbeat from the monitor, regular and reassuring.

Carl arrived at the end of his workday and labor was becoming active. We settled in for the long haul. Lights low, contractions regular, baby's heartbeat regular. In my comfort zone. All was well.

The hours started to drag, and we got a new nurse. The contractions were intense. Searing, intense, hot pain in the center of my being—and only 5 centimeters dilated. Could I make it through each one till delivery?

"I want an epidural!" The words flew out of my mouth at the height of the contraction. The nurse scurried out to get the doctor. In the calm between contractions, I looked at Carl and said, "I think I would try to talk my own patient out of the epidural at this point. It is active labor. I don't want to slow anything down."

"Whatever you want. I will help you breathe through it."

Another intense contraction, pressure, pain, dark closing around my attention, rushing in my ears. Then release. The anesthesiology resident hustled in, disheveled, sleepy from the call room.

"I'm sorry they woke you up. I'm going to do without the epidural."

"No problem."

The contractions were getting even worse. Pressure pulling my whole attention into it—dark concentrated unconsciousness—pulling me in. And then, when it was so intense that I thought I would go blind, pop! a release, as through a film or membrane, my consciousness was out of my body and watching from above. The atmosphere was pure comfort and expansiveness, like a palpable, expansive night sky. Ahhh, this is great. I can do this as long as it takes.

Time stood still, or passed, as my awareness was held in the cradle of lush heavenly energy.

And then the nurse was checking my cervix, saying, "OK. Time to push!"

That would require me to come back in my body. I don't think so. I like it up here.

"Time to push!!"

Considering coming back into the body to push. I was enjoying the comfort around me. And then, my awareness was drawn to the most attractive, sparkling light in the heavens, moving past me. I watched it move toward my body—no, toward baby Jessica's body. I followed its shining beam instinctively. Then I realized the this was Jessica's soul light committing to her body.

The soul light settled and anchored into Jessica as she moved through the birth canal. This was the perfect answer to my unspoken question: What brings the soul to the body?

My own consciousness also began to move toward my body. The part that was moving toward my body was also light. Pure being. It was my own sweet soul light. My soul awareness was coming right behind my daughter's, anchoring back into my body and pushing this baby into the world. She was being born, and I was being born new, right behind. A miracle!

The heart rate monitor was beating away, distracting my awareness for a moment—there were decelerations with every push. The cord was being compressed. Someone else would have to be concerned about that this time.

A small army of neonatology staff filed in the room and surrounded the bassinette. Extras for the doctor's baby.

A few more pushes, and Jessica was born. She was whisked over to the bassinette and she perked right up. Then she was carried back to me in someone's capable arms. The joy was palpable. The expansive heaven had descended over the entire room and enveloped all of us. This was familiar from all the births I had attended, but this was the first time I was the mother at the center of it.

It was as if my soul moved out of my body and made way for the new soul to come in to the world. Then my soul returned, but in a new way. When my daughter was born, I was also born anew into my life as a mother. I would never be the same again.

❦

Now, under anesthesia, I was feeling my soul as a watchful consciousness, ever at the ready, to bring in what awaited.

Once more, I recognized the role of surgeon went beyond the medical procedure.

A rush of power as He enters
    the shaman's zone,
        pulls the knife
          across the skin
            opens the portal
Surge of vast energy
        flowing in—

Spirit enlivens the body
    Flow /Light/Life force/ Chi

From the beginning, cells absorb it
      and become fleshy
        I am Flesh.
When the flow slows, Chi narrows
      From all the little hurts,
        Sadness walled off
          in inconvenient places—
The flesh starves,
    becomes still
      Dark
        a black hole
Until there is no flesh

Divorced from spirit, the body suffers.
The surgeon now lifts his knife
      cuts out
        black holes
Where flow can no longer reach flesh
Cuts out the sadness,

The pinched off...
Opens the channels again
    Lets the emotions flow
        Healing/Life Force
           Try again.
A trickle, a flow, a river
    Pool in the holes—fill the space
        Welling up—whetting the cells and tissues.
        New fleshy flesh.
Heart and Soul enliven me again.

Surgeon and patient.
Shaman and dreamer.

Taking the diseased, distorted,
    Walled off flesh
    That part no longer enlivened by spirit—
And cleans up
    Brings in life
        Makes it better.
Then...
    Sews it up.
        Closes the incision.
Takes off the gown, gloves, mask.
    And breathes once more ordinary air
With rational mind back.

As I watched, I saw I was the ill patient, no longer the shaman.

Terry and I had a chance to talk the day after my surgery.

"It was very cool to be 'in' the operating room, and it happened much like you said. I was poised and ready at 1:00, but was the surgery late? I felt it didn't start till 1:45."

I went silent. How did he know?

"Actually, the clock said 1:45 right before I went out."

We both smiled.

"You're amazing!" I said.

Terry went on to say that he was able to follow the surgeon, energetically restructuring the tissues as he cut. He said he sensed there were six lymph nodes removed on each side, which surprised him because I had mentioned in passing that a couple of lymph nodes might be removed from each side.

"Was that right?" Terry asked.

"Yes, you were right, Terry!" I said. "I was disappointed that the surgeon had to take so many."

"This healing had many technical aspects as I followed the surgeon doing his work. Again, I was drawn to clear your heart and reinforce the opening that you are starting to experience. This is a new way of running your heart energy, and it takes patience and tenderness to keep it open. Be sure you take your time to recover. Find time for stillness to listen to your heart. Nothing else matters now."

"Thank you, Terry. I am so grateful to have you with me on this."

As I hung up the phone, tears sprang to my eyes. I was somehow being held by him in a sacred healing space, a temple for recovery. In order to participate fully, I'd had to crack myself open. It is easy enough to open up a body with a scalpel, but not so easy to truly open one's mind and heart.

9. Dancing Heart

TWO WEEKS AFTER SURGERY, it was time for my first post-op checkup at Dr. Kinney's office. I hoped the worst was over. I'd had a lumpectomy on both breasts, and lymph node removal from each armpit. The four scars were healing well—one on each breast and one in each armpit.

As Dr. Kinney examined my breasts and my scars, I felt dread. He picked up my chart.

"The good news is that the tumor is grade 1, like we thought, and the receptors are estrogen positive and HR2 negative—the best prognosis. So that's good. The lymph node pathology shows that one node out of six on each side had a few millimeters of cancer cells. This is called micro-metastasis and it doesn't change the stage. Also, the tumor on the right extends to the edge of the specimen, so we don't have a clean margin. It appears there are runners extending past the margin.

What was he saying? There was still cancer in my body.

"So I need another surgery?"

"I'm sorry. We can do it as a day surgery case. I just need to skim the margins along one side. It won't be as extensive as the other surgery."

We scheduled another surgery, and I left the office as quickly as possible.

Safely in my car, stingy, grudging tears began to flow. *What is this, always something more? I just want it behind me!*

As the tears began to flow more freely, my body relaxed.

I heard the words: *Look deeper. Unlock the wisdom within.*

※

I was a medical student when I first recognized the OR as a sacred space between worlds. I needed to get back to that time when I was not afraid of the operating room.

I started my surgery rotation as a medical student at Rush Medical College in Chicago just to fulfill the requirement. It never occurred to me that I would become a surgeon. During the very first week, everything changed.

I was standing at the scrub sink with my resident, scrub hat and mask in place, going through the ritual of scrubbing our hands and forearms. I knew the routine now, and standing elbow to elbow with my resident, a thrill ran through me. *He's happy.* He will be the primary surgeon, and I have caught his enthusiasm. We walked into the operating room, arms up and elbows dripping. The room felt larger than usual, and my awareness was heightened. The rough towel in my hand, then the gown placed on my arms, gloves snapped onto my hands—all in rhythm with the other preparations of doctors and patient. Moving in beside my resident with my hands on the surgical field, I felt I was in the right place. As the resident pulled the scalpel along the skin to make the incision, the sky seemed to open. This entire team was holding open a sacred space for the patient. We were between the worlds.

This was the first time in medicine that I experienced the vast spirit world. I had forgotten. In surgery: That was when I realized I should become a surgeon.

Later that week, after our surgeries were done for the morning, my resident took me into the operating room where an open-heart surgery was soon to be performed. The cardiac surgeon was jovial and welcomed our presence. Perched on a tall stool behind the surgical team, I had a good view of the surgical field. A saw was used to split open the chest, and after it was cracked open, something was jumping. Incredibly, the heart was literally dancing! I never imagined that it was so active—swelling, then squeezing. I could have squealed, it made me so joyful! And the lungs were inflating and deflating in their own rhythm. Soon after, the heart and lungs quieted as the heart-lung machine took over. The remainder of the surgery was rather small, tedious, and hard to see as an observer.

I never tired of seeing the heart dancing—it seemed so perfect and impossible to me. Every time there was an open-heart surgery, I would sneak in to get a look at the dancing heart.

My obstetrics and gynecology rotation was last, because it never occurred to me that I would go into that field of medicine.

At that time in the late 70s, OB/GYN was a male-dominated profession, and the doctors seemed less academic, more surgical, and even chauvinistic. Thinking back on it all, it was suddenly so clear to me why I was drawn to this very female-oriented field of medicine...my connection to the feminine was weak in my life. I had modeled myself after my father, which was not a bad thing, but I'd dismissed my mother and her emotionality. Ironically, this was an area I needed to understand more fully and embrace in myself.

In that OB rotation, the deliveries captivated me. After a week on the rotation, it was my turn to be guided through delivering a baby. As my resident and I entered the room all gowned and gloved, we could see the baby's scalp pushing a quarter sized through the perineum. I moved between the patient's legs, in stirrups, and touched the little head with my gloved hand. Electricity moved through me. Energy was palpable in the room. *I am in the right place. This is a miracle.*

My resident guided my hands and managed all the instruments. All I had to do was hold this newborn coming from the other world to this one. I could barely think. The peace and energy in this new little person took my breath away. *I might have to do this.*

All of my carefully laid plans were being challenged. Perhaps I could become an internist, and then deliver babies, too. *Ok, that's crazy.* If I did gynecology, I could do surgery, primary care, deliver babies.

Now, decades later, finding myself in the vulnerable spot as patient due for yet another surgery, my connection with the birth process, and the essence of life energy, came flooding back to me. Sure, I was doing a good job but I'd been living my life from the neck up, cerebrally, assuming I'd figured everything out. But life and healing are not something that can be "figured out." It was coming from a very deep inner spring, and those first experiences as a young surgeon and obstetrician now flooded back to me.

The small-minded distractions of life, even in the early days, would suddenly be balanced by a vision of the eternal. It was in the middle of an argument with Carl, after I became a mother, that I was called to the hospital to be shown the big picture once again.

The conflict had grown in intensity.

"I just want more time with our girls," I was shouting.

"You became a doctor—if you didn't want to work, you shouldn't have become a doctor."

"I didn't say I didn't want to work. I want to work. I just want to work less while my kids are young. And it's ok to get paid less."

"Well, THAT'S NOT OK WITH ME! When I married you, you agreed to work full time as an OB/GYN, and now you are going back on your promise."

"I never promised you that. And I do want to work--I just want to balance my life!"

"I'm counting on you." And then, "I can fit everything into my life and work full time! You don't even manage to meet with the architect and decorator—it's not that important to you--"

"That's not fair--"

I was being a mother! I did not have much free time, but my first priority was still my kids. I got ready for bed. We turned our backs to each other in bed, anger flowing through my body. In the wee hours of the morning, I got a call from the hospital. What happened next showed me something I'd never quite seen before.

"Dr. Mitchell, we have Jeannie Walker here in active labor. Her water broke on the way here."

"Whoa! I'll be right there!"

I jumped out of bed and raced off. My fight with Carl was still a knot in my stomach. Arriving on the Labor and Delivery Unit in a rush, the nurses urged me to change into scrubs. The knot vanished; I was about to deliver a baby.

"Hurry, she is starting to push. She's been completely dilated for about 20 minutes!"

In the birthing room, the lights were low and soft music was playing. No strife. The bed had been broken down and foot rests pulled out so the patient could squat while still in the bed. The nurse stood on one side of her, and her husband on the other.

Glancing at the heart rate monitor, then at my patient, I said, "Your baby is doing very well with these strong contractions. I'd like to check you now."

I moved between her legs, pulled on a sterile gown and gloves, and inserted two fingers into her vagina. The head was descending close to the vaginal opening. She would need to push some more. I turned to prepare all the instruments on the sterile table, suction bulb for baby, clamps and scissors for the cord, basin for placenta.

We got into a rhythm—the contraction started, she pushed, I stretched out the perineum with my hands, and the head descended. Then we rested. There was a rhythm of intense effort and then relaxation.

"Ok, here we go again," I whispered. "Good. Push. You are doing it...there it comes...baby's head really moved that time... now just breathe."

Two steps forward, one step back. First babies take more pushing.

Then something extraordinary happened that I'd not quite felt as intensely before. Through this rhythm, contraction then release, an overwhelming sense of peace suddenly came over me. Time seemed to slow and the room expanded. It was as if the night sky reached down around me. Although my body was planted in the birthing room with my patient, I was part of the midnight sky, feeling the pulsation of the teeming void. The movement of this palpable energy formed into rich waves, huge folded blankets of midnight sky forming and slowly, steadily moving toward one another, coming together to form something else, something new. *Oh, this is how everything is born.* The whole manifest world is created from the enfolding of energies rising out of the void.

With my hands poised ready to receive this baby, everything was connected. In embryology, as the little embryo grows, the cells and tissues that are farthest apart come to fold over, touch together, and induce a new type of tissue or organ. The neural tube that will later become the brain and spinal cord forms from this enfolding on the microscopic level. And so it is on the vast scale of the Universe. Everything manifest comes out of the Void, and coalesces into thought and matter by this enfolding process. And every new baby being born is a representation of this process of creation. A rush of energy moved through me. *I am connected with one little baby, and the whole night sky involved in the process of creation.*

Then, the night sky receded, and I was back in the birthing room.

The baby's head was showing now—and didn't move back up with the pushing. My hand moved to cup the head, hovering, barely touching the wet scalp and hair. My other hand pushed hard on the perineal skin, holding it intact against the pressure. Holding. We pushed against each other, and the head slowly eased forward. Pop! The head was out! My left hand moved to grasp the neck from behind and support the head. As the little body shot out, my right hand maneuvered the baby's body to cradle her along my forearm. My right hand was free to suction the nose and mouth, wipe the face, rub the back. Time stood still, waiting for this baby to breathe.

And then the baby took her first big breath. Everyone took a breath. The baby cried. Then we all cried and laughed with joy.

"She's here! She is perfect," I said.

"Oh, Dr. Mitchell. She's ok?"

"Yes, she is beautiful." Looking into the baby's eyes, "Hey, Baby, welcome to the world."

Reaching to the table and finding the two clamps, I clamped them side-by-side on the umbilical cord. Then, using the scissors to cut between the clamps through the firm jelly, baby was free! Looking at the cut end of the cord, there were three blood vessels. Normal. Holding the little damp body, I lifted her up onto her Mom's tummy. She drew her baby close.

Contractions again. A rush of blood. The placenta was delivering. Placing my right hand on the abdomen and pushing down to massage the uterine fundus, left hand holding the remaining cord clamp, and gently pulling to guide the placenta out. Slowly, slowly, then pop! Into the basin. A steady rush of blood. Massaging the uterus, it contracted down and the bleeding slowed. Examining my patient, there were no tears, no cuts. Ahhh, complete.

I moved to the mother's side and slipped my arm around her shoulder, gave her a hug, and rested my other arm on hers as she held the baby—cradling Mom who was cradling her baby. Dad was next to her on the other side... We were mesmerized by this new little being. This baby had a consciousness and presence that drew us in and held us in a moment of knowing and being.

It was 4:00 in the morning by the time we finished the delivery so I decided to sleep in the call room for a few hours. That way I could make rounds on my patients.

When I awoke later that morning, a dream came back to me. Working with wood, building something with wood, picking up a handsaw, and with a slight mis-maneuver, my hand was completely severed. My right hand was cut off.

Sitting on the edge of the bed, I called Carl, who was still at home.

"Hello?"

Hearing his voice comforted me.

"Hi," I said, sheepishly.

"Mar, I had the weirdest dream last night," he said. "I never dream, but this one stood out. There was wood everywhere, it was being chopped, and my right hand got chopped off."

I was stunned. I told him I had the same dream that night.

A big silence followed.

"That's amazing," he said.

"I guess we both feel the same, that we are vital to each other. It would be like losing our right hand to lose each other," I said.

"I love you, Mar."

When we hung up, I sat in bed in the tiny call room and marveled at the previous night's experiences. During the miracle of birth, I was shown the vast world of creation; and through our dreams, Carl and I were reminded that human beings are connected to one another by something beyond any of our petty disagreements.

Over the years, navigating professional demands, family, conflict with Carl, and all the human turmoil that comes up in the course of living a life--despite it all--I always had a magical relationship with the OR. So why now was I feeling so lost, being confronted with the unexpected: I still needed more healing.

How could I tap back into that unlimited life energy?

10. The Cage

IN THE OUTPATIENT SURGERY department, I was sitting upright and cross-legged in a large recliner chair, again in my surgical gown and socks. Carl had just burst into my cubicle and was pacing around the room nervously.

"Well, if this doesn't work, Kinney said you will have to have a mastectomy. That lobular cancer sends out little runners that make it nearly impossible to get clear margins," he said.

"What? This is the first time I have heard the word mastectomy. He never said that to me."

"Well, he didn't want to upset you until he had to."

"Great." Carl always fears the worst.

After a bit, the head nurse of Outpatient Surgery came into my cubicle and said, "Dr. Wilson is tied up in the main OR and won't be free in time to do your anesthesia, Dr. Mitchell. I'm sorry." (I had made a special request for Dr. Wilson to be my anesthesiologist, but that wasn't going to be possible.)

"Dr. Walters is available," she continued.

"No! No! Not Carla Walters!" I was shocked to hear myself screeching.

The nurse stepped back and said, "OK. No problem," then quickly disappeared.

I was aware of Carl staring at me, but I looked straight ahead. Rage was coursing through me from somewhere in my depths, and I had no explanation. No proof. But he and Carla were often friendly, and she stored her car in our large garage over the winter. Some part of me knew that she did not belong in my surgery, putting me to sleep. Some part that woke up and spoke.

The nurse stuck her head back in the room, and said, "Dr. Silvers is available."

"That's great. Thank you."

Dr. Kinney arrived, and I immediately confronted him. "Carl said you might have to do a mastectomy. Is that right?"

"Whoa. We are taking another margin, that's all. Of course, if the margins aren't clear after this, that's one option. Let's just cross that bridge when we come to it."

This is a circus!

Dr. Silvers joined us. "Hi Marilyn. I'm sorry—I didn't know about the cancer."

"Hi Terry. Thanks for doing my anesthesia."

The doctors filed out, all but Carl. I was grateful when Jeannie, my 20-year friend and a pastor, came into the cubicle. She gathered my mom, Carl, and my girls around me and said a prayer for smooth, speedy, and successful surgery.

Moments later I was walking through the "No Admittance" door with my nurse and into OR # 3.

Settling into the table, I was instantly asleep.

Resting in an anesthetized state, resting in my soul. The surgeon again was standing over me. Peace. Ease. I was vast flowing energy, elevated above my body.

A question formed: Can I bring this soul energy to my body now for a new beginning? A true healing? Cancer feels more complicated than some illnesses: more insidious, pervasive, ingrained.

I became aware of something below, something between this heavenly place and my body on the operating table—an expanse of netting or grid work surrounding the body. Observing, there were multiple layers and patterns, and these grids somehow appeared to act as blinds on windows, sometimes casting shadows on the body and sometimes allowing full light. But what was the light? As my consciousness opened, I again recognized that it was my soul that was the light.

And of course! These patterns were the 9th level belief grids, representing my unconscious beliefs. Under anesthesia I was seeing it from my soul's perspective, viewing through my energy field to my own body. I needed to address these beliefs and shift them to bring more healing support to my body. A healer reinforces healthy belief grids, exchanging limiting beliefs for healing beliefs.

It was interesting to view the many concentric layers of the energy field and how much soul light they allowed through to the body. As a healer, I recognized the regular pattern of energy fields surrounding the body and how they represented different energies in our lives. As a doctor, I also knew that energy fields surround every organ, and each organ's energy exists even before it is manifested physically. Illness first happens in the field, and then comes into the body.

It was stunning to see from this perspective.

From this vantage point, a more complete knowing dawned on me: The 9th level grids move and shift like a combination lock, regulating the soul light that can come through.

This was a big revelation for me, one which I never clearly understood before. I had received an extraordinary insight.

Time passed.

Then a deep dark surrounded me. I saw a trap clamping down, holding tight, making me forget how broad and expansive I am.

The bars were made of furtive, rigid, tensile thought.

Suddenly I heard a hard voice of The Disciplinarian commanding me to "Stay in Line."

"Be productive."

"Get things done."

"Alone is best."

I had within me the knowledge of something greater, but the cancer remained. *Is there something I need to know? Please show me.*

Quiet. Relaxation. Waiting.

Then I saw it clearly. What was it?

A twisted black iron cage began to appear around my chest. As I watched, it became more clear and intricate. Feeling into it, listening. Somehow it came to me that this cage was shutting down my heart energy, containing and constricting it, and I had crafted this cage, blocking spirit.

I had not loved myself. I had been a fortress, decided early in life that I didn't need help. No one was listening to me so I stopped listening to my deeper self. I had pushed myself to be productive, to care for others, be strong and not need anything myself.

This Cage held me, lied to me that I wouldn't exist without it, hypnotized me, told me it was "real." It was a structure of habit, a protective mechanism, always on guard, tightening in, distracting me.

Release the Flow
River/Light/Essence
  so it will rise up,
      Grow
          Overflow
                Bathe
                    Overwhelm

A music came up from my heart.

I call to you, Pure Light. Let the flow start.
Flow through my dry riverbeds.
Push up from within.
Pool in my womb.
Open the floodgates.
Flow through the bars of the cage and bathe them.
Soften them to relax and let go.
Be held by the Divine Love/Light of the River flow.
Fluid, golden white warm flow.
Overflow, bathe, soothe—no boundaries
through bone and joint,
brain and eyeballs,
cell membranes and tissues
through DNA;
through the space between atoms and molecules.
Existing everywhere and flowing from the great void
and multipotent outer/inner space.
Heal me.
Unify me.
Tap the Source—not to "harness" it (as cage proposes), but
to focus—through the heart, the pelvis, then later the voice, the
brain with its pineal. Pooling, bathing, healing, collecting.
Then radiating out into life—a source of Radiance and Ecstasy.
So Be It.

As I lay in the recovery room, I saw the black cage, and again
located it around my chest. I knew that it had been crafted over
years and had locked me in. A display of scenes began to appear
on my mind screen, snapshots of my life beginning from recent
and rolling backwards until I was very young. I crafted this limited cage from an early age, adding to it through the years, forming as a mental response to difficult situations. It was crafted to
keep me "safe" from feeling my deep emotions, and to keep my

attention in my head. It was the energy representation of my mind patterns, and it had shaped my personality. Only love and tenderness for myself could melt it.

Tears of relief and compassion began to flow—for myself. I could begin to heal.

Truth with myself was key.

I closed my eyes and slowed my breath.
After some time, these words came:

Ease open the cage
    All is well.
Feeling peace, grace, and well being
      Flowing in
          Letting go of the old
Allowing the rigid cage/defense to soften
    And feeling the slow but sure
        Grace and warmth
         Growing within
Essence/Radiance
    Taking a place within me
      Being allowed to stay, grow.
The cage (made of thoughts) is fearful of annihilation/obliteration
    Without the cage, can I stand up on my own?

The next day, recovering at home, I again thought about the cage. It surprised me to realize that I had been functioning with such a split between mind and heart, especially since I had helped so many patients with this very thing. As I reflected, a tension began to well up in me. *Fear.* I was afraid to lose the support of the cage—afraid that I would be nothing without it. My mind had been my survival mechanism. Who would I be without that?

Won't it be like the bag of bones? Suddenly I remembered a recurring dream I had as a teenager. In the dream, I would be climbing the stairs in my house and stop halfway when I looked up to the landing to see my mother puddled on the floor like a bag of skin. Contained in this bag of her skin were disjointed, disconnected bones. She was unable to stand up because her skeleton was not connected.

I dreamed this dream many nights, and I thought it meant that without the structure of the mind holding things together, I would fall apart into overwhelming emotions—I would cease to exist—or be unable to walk forward and function in the world. This was represented by my mother in the dream, because my assessment was that her emotional side overwhelmed her and caused her to be ineffectual in the world.

> I must let it go gently, I've been attached to it.
> Ah, my dear survival cage:
> Trust.
> This light essence carries
> Power, verve, life force.
> It is the fuel for life and purpose
> Allow it to grow
> Nurture it
> It will then instruct your form and structure anew
> And become a container of delight, not a cage.
> A home, not a prison,
> So Be It.

It was becoming clear to me that my mind, the cage, had been my survival mechanism, seemingly keeping me "safe", but also keeping my heart from feeling—burying and storing all my emotions and longings. This shutting down blunted not only the sadness, but the joy and delight. It isn't as if I didn't understand this pattern. I witnessed it in my patients many times. I pondered the difficulty of softening the "cage of rigid thoughts" to allow the heart and soul connection to come through. I realized that it was a matter of surrender, being willing to feel the emotions. And it wasn't going to be a project that was ever finished, but a practice. Each time a wave of emotion arose, and transmuted, it made more room to breathe and live.

The cage could become a container. Softer thoughts. Creative, encouraging thoughts.

A home, not a prison.
A home.
A nest.

I was stunned. *This is true.* It can be that simple.

A wonderful sense of peace came over me. As my eyes closed, I heard the words, *The time is coming when you will be free.*

I couldn't wait to tell Terry.

11. My Father Awakens to Soul

THE FOLLOWING WEEK, I was at home recovering.

One morning, I went outside to the garden behind my house and stood by the crab apple tree to do Tai Chi. The smell was pleasant, and a calm came over me. This was the tree that my office staff had planted in honor of my father when he died. My eyes settled on the plaque placed at the base of the tree:

In Memory of Jim Mitchell
Who Saw the Divine in Nature

My feet connected with the earth, arms raised, I started the slow Tai Chi   motions, feeling a lovely surge of energy flowing through my limbs, my head, my belly. Then a sense of pure calm settled over me, and my mind was filled with a knowing, a message: *Dad is very proud of me and honors my way of being in the world. He loves me very much.* A feeling of satisfaction and connection opened within me till I felt expanded and connected with something greater.

When my cell phone rang, I knew it was Dr. Kinney. He told me the margins of tumor were clean. The most recent surgery was a success. I hung up the phone, flooded with relief, and sat back down in the garden. Gazing at my father's plaque, I found myself in a deep meditation about the nature of life and death.

When my father died sixteen years earlier, it was a shock to me. I had a glimmer of the moment when the soul separated from the body, and I realized my soul still had a decision to make.

I was at my office working when the receptionist told me I had a call from an ER in Michigan. Concern was written on her face.

What is this? Must be one of my couples—maybe premature labor? I picked up the phone.

"This is the chaplain at St. Joseph's Hospital. I'm sorry to have to tell you your parents have been in a motorcycle accident, and your father has died."

I was silent for a moment, then said, "I'm sorry, you must have the wrong person. My parents don't ride motorcycles."

"Just a moment...," the voice on the phone said. "I'm sorry. They were on bicycles. Your father died at the scene, but your mother is here in the ER. She is stable with some injuries. She doesn't know about your father yet."

I fell silent.

Then..

"Is my mom ok? What happened?"

I knew my parents were spending six weeks in a cabin in Michigan, training for a 50-mile bike ride, vacationing, and casually shopping around for a possible retirement home.

I then learned that a car had veered off the road and into the bike lane. My father was behind and he was hit first, and then my mom. For a short time, she was unconscious, but the police and ambulance arrived on the scene quickly. From the time she arrived at the hospital, she had remained conscious, and regularly asked about my Dad.

I hung up the phone, stunned. All I wanted to do was get in the car and go there. My nurse peeked her head around the door and I told her about the accident. She moved around the desk to give me a hug and reassured me that all the patients would be rescheduled.

Before I could pick up the phone, my office manager appeared in the doorway. She offered to call Carl and notify the other doctors.

I stood frozen. Time stopped. Then Carl burst in. His deep brown eyes were full of tears.

"I was making rounds. I came right away."

And then his arms were around me, holding me, and I felt my body again, aching, breathing. A sob welled up from deep in my belly. We held each other. All the issues between us disappeared, and we were connected, chests touching, hearts beating and speaking to each other.

On the three-hour drive to Michigan, Carl drove and I called the hospital to check in on my mom. The nurse's voice, on speaker, gave her report telling us that Mom was not in pain, and was stable physically. She still didn't remember the accident, as she was unconsciousness until she arrived at the hospital. They hadn't yet told her that her husband was dead.

Riding along in the car, my mind kept settling on that time right after the accident, the time my mom could not remember. Closing my eyes, I was there, witnessing the scene from above. In slow motion, the car hit my dad and his neck broke releasing his soul light from the body, which was cast aside. The light rose up, and then another light was evident, rising up. It was Mom! The souls of my mother and father lingered together in the ether, connecting, communing. My heart opened knowing that they were still connected. Although I heard no words, I knew they were communing, being together, merging for this moment before parting. He was moving on, and she was coming back. They had said their good-byes.

Why did my father leave the world? Why was my mother spared? Suddenly it hit me. The decision to live or die is, of course, not one the mind makes. That decision is a soul decision.

On some level, it seemed that Dad's soul knew of his impending death. Since the soul exists outside of time, it had a guiding effect up to the moment of his death. For one thing, he had just completed and signed his will into final form the day before they left on this vacation. And Mom also had told me about two significant events that happened the week before he died.

They had gone to the beach, and Dad decided to wade out into the waves while my mom observed on the shore. As she watched, Dad went out into the waves, laughing and playing like a child. She saw him become one with the rhythm and play of the tide. Time stopped. At that moment, it struck her at the time as something important, but later as she recalled this moment, she felt that he was connecting to the place he would inhabit days later.

Another evening, after dinner, Dad lay down to stretch his back. This was a routine he had for years. He would lie down on the bed and stretch his achy back for a few minutes before returning to the kitchen to help my mom with the dishes. Four days before his death, he went once more to lie down on the bed. Mom did all the dishes, wiped the counters, turned out the light in the kitchen, and went into the bedroom. Dad was sleeping more deeply than she had ever remembered. It got her attention because it was so different. He slept in the same exact spot until the following morning. She thought that he must have made a brief journey to heaven.

We arrived at the hospital and we were whisked right in, past reception, past the "No Admittance" sign, past the ER nurses station. The nurse pulled back the curtain from bed #2. Mom. She was on a gurney with her head upright. Her eyes locked onto mine.

"Oh, Honey! Dad is gone," she said. So they had finally told her.

I walked forward and we embraced. Carl moved right behind me and took my mom's hand. Without looking at him I felt him crying. Helpless. We were in our own cocoon, the three of us, as Mom told us what she remembered: on their bicycles on Red Arrow Highway (in the bike lane); only had a short stretch to go on the old road; she was in front, Dad behind; the last thing she remembered was seeing the Antique Barn up ahead on the right where they had planned to stop for a break.

The curtain whooshed open, and the young ER doctor burst in. After introducing himself and checking how my mom was feeling, he began to tell us about her injuries, and her current status. Strange how comforting it was to hear this medical report doctor-to-doctor. He clearly wanted to do something for us, and this was what he could offer. Mom had a foot injury, broken ribs, a fractured pelvis, and multiple scrapes and bruises. The doctor then took us to the X-ray view box to show us the broken ribs. She would need to be observed overnight with cardiac monitoring. Mobile ribs can sometimes cause the heart to be affected. The doctor was amazed that Mom was not experiencing more pain.

My world was now turned upside down. My dad was gone and my heart was thrown wide open to my mother. No more guarding my heart from her. So this is it: the end of my Dad's earthly story. I didn't know till that moment that I had assumed my mom would go first, and my dad and I would someday have the luxury of time to share life again. With my mom out of the way...He would live with me in his older age, perhaps. But now that had all changed. The connection to my mother was now open and I just wanted to protect her--scoop her up and take her home. I was about to get to know her.

Remembering this, I was hit with another realization. By guarding against my mother for so long, I'd also blocked my access to the spirit of the divine feminine. Now, in my healing, I had more work to do on that.

Later that day at the hospital, the police officers filled in a few more details: the driver was an 83-year-old woman whose driver's license was expired. She was driving her grandson somewhere and had an obstructed view due to the sun in her eyes, or the grandson having a newspaper open. In any case, she swerved off the road. The officers explained that Michigan is a no-fault state when it came to traffic accidents, and even though my parents were on bicycles and not in a car, their car insurance would be taking care of expenses. The officers wanted to know if we were going to press charges against the driver. One officer said this was ultimately up to my mom, and we didn't have to decide right away. He had my father's belongings and would bring them to me later.

Back with my mom in the ER cubicle, I was struck with a strong urge to see my dad. I pulled back the curtain and walked up to the nurse at the desk.

The chaplain was sitting vigil with the nurse. Walking up to them, I leaned over the counter and with my most winning smile, and firm but kind doctor's voice, I said, "I want to go see my dad in the morgue. My husband wants to come, too."

Shock came over their faces. "We've never done that."

"Don't worry," I said. "We are both doctors, and besides, it is not uncommon to go to the morgue when a baby dies. We routinely offer this to the parents so they can see and hold their babies."

"Hmmm. Let me see what I can find out," the nurse said.

I walked back into my mom's cubicle and told her what I had requested. She wanted to go, too.

A half hour later, we had an entourage winding through the hospital halls toward the morgue: Carl, me, Mom being pushed on the gurney by a nurse, the chaplain, and the two policemen who had been standing by. It was a coroner's case because of the accident. We all crowded onto the service elevator going down.

At the basement level the elevator doors opened, and we saw a room that said "No Admittance." We all exited the elevator and waited outside the room.

After five minutes, a man in a lab coat came out of the room. Carl, my mom and I were allowed to go in. He opened the door, and as I walked through, I saw my dad on a steel table. *This is where they will do the autopsy.* The room looked somewhat like an operating room, tiled, with steel sinks, and lights above the table. Walking over to my dad, a peaceful feeling came over me. Nothing surreal. My eyes scanned his clothes, his face, his body—no scars, no evidence of trauma—just him, very still. He had been laid here as if he were sleeping, nothing out of order. *It is definitely his body, but he is not here.* My mind struggled to understand this, but something deep in me was satisfied. He was a free soul now. I became aware of Carl across the room, and his sadness. We wheeled my mom closer to my father's body.

"Oh, Jim," she wept. "Why didn't you take me with you?"

I put my hand on her shoulder. "I know, Mom, but I'm glad you are still here. I wasn't meant to lose both my parents at once."

When we returned to the ER we learned that they were ready to transfer my mom to a monitored hospital bed. Carl and I decided to go to the police station to collect my Dad's belongings and then go to the cabin where they were on vacation, to pack it up.

While we were packing, Carl and I changed out of our work clothes into my parent's casual clothes. Carl donned my father's shorts, a T-shirt, and topsiders. One of the best influences in his life had been my father. All strife between us was now gone. We seemed to be inhabiting an expansive type of soul bubble. I had wanted that to last forever.

I loved that Carl kept those same clothes for many years, wearing them regularly to work outdoors in the garden.

∽

I alerted all my friends and family that my breast surgeries were successfully completed. Still, I sensed a deep shift was required for me to fully restore my life energy. What I'd really been up to all this time, I realized, in my healing practice, was connecting my patients to a deep desire to live, a soul desire. I needed to do that for myself.

12. A Cardinal for Aunt Bettie

How do your access your own soul? The truth was I didn't know how.

Signs of spring were beginning to show; birds returned from their winter break in the south and often stopped to explore our yard. It was a nice place for nesting, with nine partially wooded acres and two ponds. I spotted a bright red cardinal day after day around the house.

Now there was a peck, peck, peck on the window, and when I went to look, it was again my cardinal friend, sitting in the tree outside. On closer inspection, I spotted his muted brown-grey mate on a nearby branch of the tree. It looked like they might have been building a nest.

Aunt Bettie! I'd almost forgotten. The last time I saw a cardinal doing this was years ago when Aunt Bettie was so sick. The cardinal was Aunt Bettie's favorite bird, and had become her symbol. Before she got sick, she was living in the house my grandfather built situated on the Fox River in Oswego, Illinois. Cardinals and other birds were abundant in that yard, visible through the big picture window at the back of the house. A huge grassy yard rolled down to the Fox River bank. Inside her house, there were cardinal artifacts everywhere—mostly gifts she had received from her family.

Aunt Bettie was my favorite aunt and had been my confidant and champion my whole life. She was 79, my mom's older sister by seven years. She was witty, fun, wise and much more relaxed and open minded than my mom. She always made me feel special, and we had many poignant moments and deep conversations. She took me seriously and made me feel that my ideas were on equal terms with hers. My mom was more strict and conservative, but she looked up to her older sister, so if Aunt Bettie talked to her about changing her mind, Mom would cut some slack and listen. Aunt Bettie came to my rescue on many occasions.

One time when I was eleven, Aunt Bettie was driving me back from my cousins' house to my grandfather's house. It was just the two of us in the car. Instead of driving straight home, she turned down the little Main Street in Oswego and into a parking place in front of the drug store. She put the car in park but left it running.

"Wait here. I just have to run in for a quick minute," she said.

It was already dark outside and there were snow flurries. I tried to watch her, but she got swallowed up as she walked to the back of the store. After five minutes, I could see her at the register, and soon after she was opening the car door and climbing in. She slammed the door and reached over to me, handing me the small brown bag with her purchase.

"This is for you."

"Me?" I thought she was picking up some aspirin or something for herself. I unrolled the top of the little brown bag and peered in.

"Wow! It's a razor!"

"Yes. You need one, don't you?" There was a smile in her voice.

"Yes, but did you talk to my mom?" Mom and I had been fighting about this for months. I had wanted to start shaving my legs, but she argued that I was not old enough.

"Yes, it's fine."

So, Aunt Bettie had worked her magic once again!

My brother later told me that when he and his friend visited Aunt Bettie on a break from college, they got her to try smoking pot with them. ("Don't tell my kids," she said.) They even left her a little joint as a souvenir, which she kept hidden in her underwear drawer. She never smoked it, and one time later in her life when she could no longer climb the stairs without getting winded, she whispered to me, "Run upstairs and get that marijuana out of my drawer before your mother takes the laundry up. She wouldn't understand."

Aunt Bettie was a nurse, and when I started med school she was very proud. She called me "little doctor" and when I was home on break, we had even more in common. She was from the old school and was one of the ones who wore nurses' caps and used "doctor" as a proper name (as in: "Doctor will see you now"). She had been an army nurse, an office nurse, a hospital nurse, an elder care nurse. Her wisdom and knowledge were vast. She was a nurse who kept doctors on track while not letting on to them. When I decided to do an OB/GYN residency, she just couldn't relate. Not her cup of tea. She liked things neat. The messiness and unpredictability of delivering babies she couldn't relate to. ("Oh, Honey. Really? How can you like that?")

Aunt Bettie was really a hoot and could be irreverent at times. When my father died suddenly and the family gathered, Aunt Bettie made her famous brownies. I came around into my kitchen to find her and my brother standing over the pan of brownies—my brother was doubled over with laughter, weeping.

"What is going on?" I asked with feigned sternness.

My brother wiped his eyes, then pointed a serving knife at Aunt Bettie for emphasis. "She said she decided to make these brownies half male and half female. When I asked what she meant, she said the male ones have nuts."

I think Aunt Bettie might have had a little Zen in her. She recognized it was best to have an equal share of maleness and femaleness, even in a brownie.

Aunt Bettie was totally herself at all costs.

It was in 2005 she informed me she had lung cancer.

She was willing to come to my hospital and see doctors I chose for her. We struggled with whether to pursue aggressive treatment, or just institute palliative measures. My oncologist colleagues assured me that there were many advances in lung cancer therapy, and it was no longer the death sentence it had been when I was in medical school, so Aunt Bettie went forward with two strenuous surgeries. (At the time, I didn't know what I know now about energy healing.) Her surgeries were probably too strenuous. The cancer progressed anyway.

Aunt Bettie and I had many discussions about where she wanted to go for care when she was discharged from the hospital. She loved her home on the river, and I offered to research hospice there. In the end she decided she wanted to be in a nursing care facility in the area where my mom and I lived. This was a place where she would feel settled, being cared for in a hospital type setting the way she had cared for so many others.

Around the time she was transferred there from the hospital, I noticed a cardinal on my property. He would often peck on different windows of my house.

As a busy doctor, it was hard to find the time to visit Aunt Bettie, except on the weekends when I was not on call. One Sunday morning, my eyes sprung open before my alarm. *I get to visit Aunt Bettie today.* The twilight feeling between waking and sleeping stayed with me as I climbed out of bed and walked out of the bedroom. When I got to the landing at the top of the stairs, I heard the familiar peck, peck, peck and looked up to see my cardinal. It made me smile, even though he pecked on a window most days since he moved in over a month earlier.

As I walked down the stairs, there was again a peck, peck, peck on the window halfway down the stairs. He had flown over the roof to the other side now. I continued my descent to the back foyer and started down the hall toward the family room. Peck, peck, peck. He had again flown to the other side of the house and was pecking at the window by his nest. *He's following me!* My gait slowed, but I made my way through the family room to the kitchen. Walking up to the kitchen sink I saw the cardinal come right up to the window facing me and peck, peck, pecking on the beveled glass! What was going on here? I hurriedly walked from the kitchen, through the butler's pantry, down the hall, and turned into the laundry room. Making a bee-line for the door, I opened it and walked out onto the stoop. I saw my bird by the kitchen window, and just said aloud "What?"

He flew off, across the back rock garden, and perched in a tree branch above the waterfall. He was staring at me. Again I asked, "What is it?" Silence. We must have stayed like this for twenty minutes. At the same instant, he flew from the branch and I turned to go back in the house.

Later that afternoon, my mom and I went to visit Aunt Bettie. She was in a single room, and when we walked in she was asleep in the hospital bed. I walked over and sat down on her bed.

"Aunt Bettie?" I said, touching her on the arm.

Her eyes shot open and looked directly into mine.

"Oh, I'm still here?"

"Were you dreaming?"

She shook her head adamantly.

"Well, tell me about it. Where were you?"

Silence. She was looking at me but had no words.

I knew she was halfway to the other side, but I sensed that it was too much effort for her to explain to me.

My mom moved closer and I got up from the bed. We talked to her, but she remained silent. She continually changed position from lying down to seated, to standing with assistance for a moment. She was restless and couldn't get comfortable. After about an hour, my mom decided to take a little break and go out in the hallway.

Aunt Bettie was sitting on the side of the bed, and I moved in to sit beside her, shoulder to shoulder. We were in a cocoon of peaceful energy, just being together. And then she turned her head, looked me straight in the eyes, and said, "That's where I want to go."

"You mean where you were when I woke you up?"

She nodded.

"It's ok to go there, but you have to wait till your kids get here."

Silence.

"Hey, do you hear me? It is ok to go. You just have to wait till your kids come. I will call them. Will you wait till they get here?'

Nodding and a direct look in my eyes. *She understands.*

When my mom came back to the room, I told her of our communication, and later that day we called her three children. They arrived the next day. Two days later, Aunt Bettie's children stood at her bedside as she lay quietly. She hadn't opened her eyes or spoken in a while. Suddenly, she opened her eyes slightly and quietly announced, "I'm outa here!" Moments later she died.

My cardinal and his family remained in my yard for the rest of the season.

⌒∽⌒

The following year on the anniversary of Aunt Bettie's death, a cardinal again came peck, peck, pecking at my windows.

Every Christmas season a cardinal would come and sit for an hour framed in my family room window so I could see him from the kitchen sink.

As I pondered how one accesses one's own soul, I realized I'd known how all along. It was all around me, connecting with nature and the spirits of loved ones through a courier between the worlds, Aunt Bettie's cardinal.

13. Oncologist

IT WAS WITH RENEWED spirit that I made plans to see an oncologist. My journey with cancer was far from over.

Dr. Holzman's office was in an ordinary suburban medical building. As I sat in the waiting area, my strong aversion to chemotherapy was kicking in. I was confident at least I could avoid that, given that my cancer was low grade and had not metastasized. I was certain also that there were alternative therapies I could use.

Sitting in the waiting area, I wasn't so sure I had all the answers. I needed to talk this over with the oncologist. I didn't want to skip steps, or try to treat myself, but I had to have doctors who were open to the alternative practice I intended to use. How did I know he would listen to me?

"Marilyn Mitchell?" a medical assistant called my name.

Following her down the hallway we reached a doorway, and she stopped and motioned for me to go in. "You can sit here in one of these chairs. The doctor will be here in just a minute."

I took a chair facing the large desk and waited.

When Dr. Holzman appeared in the doorway, I remembered I'd just seen him a few weeks earlier at a reception my medical practice had thrown for colleagues.

"Hi there," he said. "I'm sorry to have to see you here."

It is difficult for doctors to treat doctors. We feel fallible and vulnerable when we are facing another doctor with an illness. We are surprised that knowing medicine doesn't protect us from getting sick.

"Well," he continued. "I have read all your records. You have Stage 1 grade 1 tumors, Her2 negative and ER-positive receptors."

I knew this meant the tumor has estrogen receptors.

"That is the best possible category. Chemotherapy isn't recommended, but low dose radiation is," he said.

I was relieved. Radiation didn't concern me. That was a vibration that I knew could be buffered with energy healing.

"You know," Dr. Holzman added, "with the estrogen positive status, you need to take an aromatase inhibitor."

Aromatase inhibitors are medications that block estrogen receptors.

A pit formed in my stomach and grew to encompass my whole body. *No!* That was out of the question! My reaction surprised me. How is it that radiation was no big deal to me, but taking the medication seemed impossible?

Aloud I said, "Is that absolutely necessary?"

"Well, in your category, taking the aromatase inhibitor has been shown to significantly reduce the recurrence of cancer."

Clearly, he thought this was a no-brainer.

"But what about the side effects? My patients all have them. I don't really want to get menopause symptoms and osteoporosis."

"We can give medications to help with that. It improves the outcome, so you have to weigh the risk/benefit ratio."

He was kind, but it was clear that he didn't understand my resistance.

"How long would I take it?" I asked, already knowing the answer.

"At least five years, based on the studies, but you don't need to start it until the radiation is done. So you can write the prescription for yourself, or I am happy to do it. Call me if you want me to prescribe after you have finished the radiation therapy."

"OK, I will," I lied.

Later, after I left the office and was driving home, I thought about the medication again. Again, the feeling of dread grew from the pit of my stomach till it involved my whole body. I started to cry, then sob. Every cell in my body was saying NO! Finally, I settled down. It was odd that the least invasive treatment in this whole process was triggering such a violent reaction.

I will find another way, and I can wait to think about it until my radiation is finished, I decided.

When I got home, I settled into my meditation chair, closed my eyes, and these words came:

Love myself...
    Open my heart to
The Flow of Love
Relax
    Deepest relaxation
    Letting go
No tense smiles
    No sweeping under the rug
Pure letting go
    Of all the tense cage
And with the holding surrendered
    Power/Light /Ecstasy flows in

Pure being
    Love—Divine Mother Love
        Love from the earth and within
        Rising up and filling up
            Filling in

So all the spaces are loved
    And find presence and substance
A loving caress and filling
    Massaging then absorbing
    Between the muscle fibers
        Deep into the fiber
            Becoming the fiber
And deeper into the cells and tissues
    Between the cells
        All the way
            Into the space between the molecules
              Inner and outer space
        Of pure potential.
All is possible.
All is well.

❧

I opened my eyes and thought, *My cells don't want the aromatase inhibitor. They want love to caress them.*

A little later, I began an Internet search. Although aromatase inhibitors were widely used and studied, I was wary of their effects. I knew of research on an alternative: a product that was an extraction from cruciferous plants. I reviewed the studies: this substance blocked estrogen receptors selectively, particularly those on breast cancer cells, while sparing receptors on other cells. That was great news for me: a product that would comply with medicine and have fewer side effects.

My cells would thank me for this: a vehicle to distribute love.

14. Radiation consult

THE GOOD SHEPHERD OUTPATIENT radiation facility was just five minutes from my house so it seemed the logical place for me to receive therapy. Dr. Kinney, my surgeon, supported my decision to go ahead with radiation, and recommended Dr. Ruffer.

Some people have a fear of the side effects or the invasiveness of radiation. But when I learned that I was a candidate for lumpectomy and radiation, I was relieved. Since radiation is an energy vibration, I reasoned, energy healing seemed like the perfect treatment to combine with it. It would be a buffer to protect the healthy cells and zap the cancer cells. Besides, several of my healing colleagues simultaneously applied energy healing to patients while they were undergoing radiation.

The medical objective of radiation after lumpectomy is to send a signal to the cells in the breast that are beginning to turn abnormal but are not detectable yet. It is said that the "field," in this case the whole breast, is a fertile ground for growing cancer, so this entire area is treated with a low dose of radiation to prevent recurrence.

After checking in, I was ushered into an exam room, where a nurse practitioner took my history, and then asked which arm she needed to avoid for taking my blood pressure. Ugh. That's right. The arm on the side of the lymph node sampling is avoided for blood pressure readings. I was still absorbing it all.

"I had bilateral surgery, but my surgeon approved me for blood pressure in both arms."

Because I am a doctor? I wondered. Hmmm. No matter. *I am going to be a special case.*

The nurse handed me a gown and left the room so I could change. Soon I would meet Dr. Ruffer. I wished I could have met him with my clothes on instead of a baby blue gown. I wanted him to meet me first as a person, not a patient. I personally met all my new patients with their clothes on.

Dr. Ruffer opened the door and instantly a warm energy put me at ease.

"Doctor," he smiled, almost teased, the way he said the word. "I am sorry we are meeting like this."

He proceeded to review my history, and then asked a few questions about my work and family to get to know me. I learned that he had four kids, his wife was a professor, and he was part of Lutheran General Group but was in charge at this facility at Good Shepherd Hospital.

He was a nice guy. Now we had a fix on each other. We were going to get along well.

"I need to examine you," he said.

There was seriousness in his tone now, a focus, to move us beyond the awkwardness. Awkward because I was not just a patient, but a female doctor who examines women routinely, and he had to touch my breasts. And then, too, because I am a doctor, this cancer case was a little too close to home.

When the exam was finished, Dr. Ruffer asked me to get dressed and meet him in the conference room to talk.

Our discussion was very helpful. Dr. Ruffer explained the procedure: I would return for measurements and tattoo marking the following day, and then a schedule of treatments would be determined, probably 5-10 minutes every weekday for six weeks. He patiently answered my numerous questions.

And then he said something I would never forget:

"Marilyn, let me tell you how it works: the healthy cells have a much higher vibration than the cancer cells. Our physics has become so much more precise in recent years that the level of radiation can be set precisely so that it will destroy cancer cells, but low enough that normal cells will still be able to recover."

That sounded like energy healing talk, not physics or medicine!

This was the first time I learned that healthy cells had a higher energy vibration than cancer cells. I didn't know it was measurable.

What a great message to keep in mind—I would tell all my healers so they could use this information when doing healings.

Walking out to my car, I felt upbeat. I have the right doctor with the right attitude!

And then it hit me: for thirty days I would be starting my day with radiation treatments. My "no big deal" approach was being challenged. I felt heavy, sad. How could I turn this into a positive?

Terry would be doing energy healings, but how would I deal with this dread that was rising in me?

Then it hit me! Why didn't I shift this into what I wanted? I could consider the radiation center a true healing center and have a healing every time I had a treatment. Since I had to prepare to be on the radiation table every morning at 7:00, I vowed to turn the same time into a daily healing.

At home, as I approached my meditation room I felt a wave of energy pass through me, followed by the thought: *I had two breast tumors, not one.*

Stopping in my tracks, I wondered: *What does this mean for me? There is something here.*

I continued down the hall to my meditation room and settled into my chair, pondering. As I relaxed, a wave of pleasant energy again passed through me. What was this wave? I realized for the first time: *This is how my soul gets my attention!*

I relaxed and let go into meditation.

Around my heart, the cage became apparent, but different, it had changed. Instead of a rigid grid, it was more ephemeral and elusive, more flexible. My heart expanded from within, and I realized I was breathing easier.

The cage was softening, transforming.

Next, in the field around my chest, the image of two tumors emerged, energy representations of the tumors that had been physically removed.

What did they have to tell me?

Both were gray-black, but the one from my right breast was larger, denser. The center felt stagnant; I sensed that energy had not reached this center in a long time. Moving closer to the periphery, there was gradually more activity—cellular activity. This tumor had been crafted over the years, slowly advancing its limits, pulling cells into the black hole of stagnation. It felt like loneliness.

My attention moved to the left tumor—smaller, lighter. The activity was slow, cells abnormal, but still alive in the center. It started more recently.

What does this mean for me? Why an old and a new tumor?

Quiet. Peaceful. Sinking in. Feeling in.

Feeling the energetic tumors, I understood that when the breast cells stopped thriving, it was because the flow of soul energy dwindled. Somehow when I had stopped listening to myself, the flow of energy stopped to my own cells. The black cage around my heart had impacted my breasts, the cage crafted from hard thoughts and suppressed emotions.

Reeling. Emotion welling inside. The tumors started from specks, a few cells not getting love. These cells coalesced and grew into tumors from my refusal to listen to my heart and connect my soul to Source Love directly. How could I be so cruel and withholding to myself?

After some moments, a wave of peace ran through me.

Soothing, comforting.

Paying attention.

Energy flowing again.

Soul here now.

Basking in the new flow, the tumors, although faded, remained and again drew my attention. Something more here. Both of these tumors were initiated from a time when love had been taken away, and I didn't listen. The larger older tumor was initiated when my marriage began to lose connection; the smaller recent tumor was initiated in a more recent loss where the love flow had been strong, and then abruptly shifted. In both cases, I had coped by shutting down my emotions and functioning from my mind, the cage. I had abandoned my heart.

Gentle tears began to come. Relief. And then the words:

I am vast—
    Ahh, I had forgotten...
I can connect
    With Love
        Source
           Flow
Even when another is cut off
    And afraid
        And their darkness pulls at me

Extending vast Love flow
I am the flow
"Nothing can separate me from the love of God."
Grace
    descend
    Be with me

Flow through my body
    Open my love and peace
Flow through my head, eyes, jaw
        Through my sadness
                Aloneness
Burst up through my heart like a fountain.
Peace in the land—
        In the terrain of my body
Even in the midst of upset others
Be the River that flows around the stressed ones
        bringing soothing water
                to their island shores.
Being peace, flow, love.

15. Radiation Healing Treatment

ON THE SHORT DRIVE to my fist session of radiation, I listened to soothing chanting music. In the small changing room, after donning my gown, I grabbed the key to my locker and my iPod. I had recorded a healing meditation to listen to during the treatment, giving my body direction about how to absorb the radiation and have a healing from it. The technician ushered me down the hall.

I'm walking to the healing treatment room, I told myself.

We walked into the room and she helped me onto the table, adjusting me into position. *This is my healing table.*

As I started to put in my ear buds, the technician said, "We have music in the room, whatever you like."

'Oh, thanks. This is a special recording I made for healing. It tells my body what I want it to do with the radiation."

"OK." She lit up. "Let me help you."

We found a spot for the iPod by my head so it wouldn't get radiated. Lying flat on the table with my chest exposed, the technicians reached up to grab the two large four-foot metal canisters that loomed over me and maneuvered them until they were pointed to just the right spot. They checked and double-checked. Then, when the positioning was exact, they left the room to administer the radiation, watching me from a control booth with a glass window. In my case they would radiate one breast, take a break to move the canisters, then vacate the room again to radiate my other breast.

My recording started as they positioned the canisters for the first time. Soothing. I closed my eyes and music played in my ears. My body relaxed into the table. Distant sounds: Click, whoosh, lock. The machines were in place and the technicians moved away from my side and left me alone in the room. Through the earphones, my voice started speaking, giving a message to my body to enjoy this healing. I thanked the cancer for getting my attention. I had heard the message, and now it was time for the cancer cells to leave. I asked the radiation to transmute those cancer cells, and I asked the healthy cells to be immune from the radiation and to recover quickly. I sent healing light to each organ and system by name.

Time to heal
    Breathe, relax
    Every tissue, every cell
        Prepare for healing
Peace, love and gratitude abound
Bathe in the rose light that permeates this healing space,
    this healing center,
            with loving attendants, physical and spirit

Open to this therapy with its sacred precision
        Radiating energy toward cancer cells
I call to you, Cancer cells:
    Absorb this radiation beam
        Allow it to gently,
            Step by step,
        Return you to the Light.
                ✐
Protect healthy cells as they
    Absorb healing light

Energize and protect
    All cells and tissues
        With peace and calm
            Feel the joy of healing.

Deeply align,
    Cancer cells, let go
        Return to Light
I have heard your message and
    Thank you
        You are released

I take deep rest and refreshment for my body
        Relaxation
           Calm
Breasts
    Rejuvenate
      Clear
        Fill with Light
          Better than before
Mind
    Peaceful
Lymphatics
    Cleared
      Stimulated
        Flow sparkling love through your channels
All is well

All my body, receive
    Energy
      Healing
Soothing energy salve abounds
    No harm done.

Go from this healing with
> Peace
>> Energy
>>> Confidence
>>>> Radiance

So Be It

As I listened, I could feel the expansion and peace of the healing energy traveling through my body. Ahhh. The recording ended just when the techs were moving the machines away. Perfect timing. The technicians pushed the canisters away and helped me off the table. I was then ushered back to the changing room.

Terry and I connected on the phone the following day. I was bursting with my insight about the two tumors and how they grew.

I felt Terry listening and was comforted by his present and reliable tone. It reflected his consistent, healing attention toward me.

"You are doing great healing because you are listening to your heart. Your healing is very important to the world and this insight you had about your cancer is profound information, for you and for others," he said.

In truth, since my diagnosis, my soul had been gently guiding and nudging me to reconnect with it. I was moved when I reflected on the beautiful meditations, significant memories, and healing relationships that were being presented to me. I had opened my heart, the gateway to my soul.

This was my soul at work, calling to me.

Soul presence.

All is well.

⁓

My second day of radiation was a Friday, the last day of that week. The routine started out the same: climb onto the table, position the iPod and earphones, then play the recording while the technicians handle the radiation part of my healing. Only today, as my mind was quiet and the recording was nearing the end, the peaceful feeling faded a little. A tense sensation rose through my body. I realized it was the cells/the body talking to me: "This is very difficult what you are asking." My heart sank. Uncertainty. *Well, I have the weekend off.*

On Sunday, I had a healing scheduled with Terry, again a distance healing. After explaining the message from my body as we talked before the healing, he said, "Let's see what we learn from the healing. We will try to keep you out of fear."

After hanging up the phone, I settled into my bed, and the familiar flow of energy began, signaling that Terry had started the healing. I drifted off, and an hour later woke right up. *He's done.*

This time Terry called me. "The most amazing thing happened," he said. "While I was working in your field, a grid started to float down for me to put in place. I knew it was a very high vibration, higher than I had ever used before. My intuition called it the 440 Grid. It is really the most incredible vibration! I have never seen anything like it."

This was a complete mystery. Neither of us knew what a 440 Grid was.

"As the grid descended down over your body," Terry explained, "it was apparent that it was in the form of your breasts. It hovered high above the body and I restructured the breasts at this high level, and when the restructuring was complete, it was as if the high vibrational breasts just flowed down to your physical body, melded with the breasts, and then expanded this energy through the chest, and finally throughout your entire body."

It seems healers are often participating in a mystery they themselves don't always understand. Some might call us mystics; our visions might seem strange or mystifying, and our role is just to see what's there.

Shivers started running through me. I understood that this cancer journey of mine had the potential to benefit many others. After a long silence, I said, "Terry, I'm not sure what this is. But you brought in something new."

Terry quietly said, "Let's see what happens if each day when you are on the radiation table, you ask for the 440 grid to descend over you."

Tears welled up. Gentle waves of energy flowed through my body. Awareness settled in: This 440 grid is another vehicle to assist soul to flow into the body.

My next radiation session was the following day, on Monday, and after settling into the table with my headphones for a healing, a wonderful rush of energy moved through me. I asked that the 440 grid descend over my body, and felt a deep, pleasant sensation starting in my chest and moving over my entire body. Expanded, my body limits were blurred.

The healing was effortless, and as the recording was ending, a wave of pleasant energy again moved through me. It was my body saying, "Much easier. We can do what you ask now."

As I left the dressing room at the radiation facility, I began to think about how I had to start relaxing my resistance to confronting cancer. *I have cancer, but I trust that after I am healed, I will not have it any more.* I had resisted the word "survivor"; to me it implied being a victim after having fought a battle. I wanted to embrace this experience for having listened to the integrative process of healing that flows when my mind/body/spirit are united, not walled off and separate. I knew I could be better than before...not just surviving. As I walked into the hall-way toward the reception area to exit, something stopped me. For years, I resisted the message of the American Cancer Society and others that use "fight" and "battle" and "survivor" language. It just seemed to escalate fear. The idea of running a campaign for "the cure" seemed a misnomer to me. True, fundraising campaigns have been enormously successful in supporting the development of more effective and humane therapies, but this was treatment, not cure. My mind was on a soapbox now about what cancer was all about, and how our language about cancer keeps us from developing a new understanding.

Why would a body form cancer, anyway? And why more and more frequently in these modern times?

Somehow, life force gets pinched off.

As I walked out into the daylight, a calm came over me. An opening. There was no need to resist the ACS or others who are "fighting" to eradicate cancer. After all, their hearts and intentions are in the right place, and in the end they wanted the same thing that I wanted. Better and safer treatments are a good thing. I walked across the parking lot, and my heart and mind felt ease.

I smiled to myself and realized: resistance is a mind ploy. All resistance is a way of blocking emotion and blocking soul flow, preventing a new understanding.

My struggle, and my healing from cancer, must move from trying to "spirit it away" and toward being fully authentic and in truth with myself. That meant releasing the mind's resistance, with its well-grooved ideas, and fully absorbing my diagnosis, treatments, emotions, all—not sliding over the surface. Quieting my mind, releasing the cage. Feeling it all. That is when the true healing and the true gifts come forth, and when I become fully alive and happy.

Being fully engaged in this journey of cancer may light a path to cure.

Grace

Grace descending
   As Chi flowing through me.
      Transforming my body
         Transforming my life
Open all the little creaks in my life.
   Light, love, Divine.

16. Yoga — connecting soul to body

YOGA HAS ALWAYS BEEN a wonderful and mindful way of exercising for me, but I had no idea how important it would become as a gateway to my healing.

Four weeks after my second surgery, I returned to a yoga immersion I'd been to before, with Chad, a yogi who reminded me of a leprechaun gymnast, or a celestial taxi driver with ADD. Another unlikely shaman. He channeled his hyperactivity with yoga and meditation. His enthusiasm was never curbed.

Walking into his studio, a calm came over me. Safe. Chad knew about my diagnosis and asked if I wanted to tell my classmates. I pondered a moment. Of course. These eight people were part of what made this place safe and peaceful.

We gathered in our circle to start our day, sitting cross-legged, and started with the invocation chant:

OM
Namah Shivaya Gurave
(I open my heart to the power of Grace)
Saccidananda Murtaye
(That lives in us as goodness)
Nisprapancaya Shantaya
(That never is absent and radiates peace)

Niralambaya Tejase
(And lights the way to transformation)
Om

Opening my eyes after the chant, the silence was palpable, pulsating. *I am in the perfect place now.* All is well.

Chad reminded us that this immersion was about "Awakening the Heart of Transformation," and then he asked what had transpired in the student's lives. After a few people spoke, it was my turn.

"Well, I had surgery for breast cancer."

Shock. Fear. All eyes riveted on me.

"It's ok. It isn't very serious," I continued. Then I heard myself saying, "It is causing me to think seriously about my relationship with myself."

A few minutes later when we moved to put out our yoga mats, everyone seemed to find a way to bump into me with a hug.

Unexpected tears. I'm not that good at being vulnerable.

The morning progressed with Chad giving a lecture on the "subtle body" anatomy—he spoke of kundalini, chakras, nadis, and koshas. The ancient tradition of yoga has taught the subtle energies for thousands of years. In my training as a healer, I'd known about chakras and auric fields, which were similar to the koshas, but I had not had experience with kundalini. It especially captivated me.

Late in the morning, the time came for our asana practice: the series of postures, movement, and breath that make up the core of yoga. We lined up our yoga mats on either side of the room, and each took our places standing at the front end of our mats facing the center of the room. Following Chad's direction, we placed our hands in prayer position at the heart, then reached to the sky to stretch, then bowed into a forward fold, then into plank position, lowered down into cobra pose, and finally, downward dog, stretching arms and legs down to the floor from the pelvis high in the air.

With each series of moves, Chad would remind us, "Follow the breath."

Breath led every move, and infused muscle and movement with life. The word "inspire" comes from the Latin "inspirare" meaning to breathe, inflame, or blow into; it has come to mean "to fill with heart or grace" or "animate with an idea or purpose." Inspiration! The yogis teach that when we breathe, we take in not only air, but also Prana or life force itself.

"Engage muscular energy. Feel it. Then feel the organic expansion—Shine Out."

Chad—a short, very muscular figure with a large balding skull—moved around us in a dance, calling out the moves, encouraging us and adjusting our postures. We moved through series after series of postures, feeling the energy grow and release, again and again, as we all moved in unison.

As I moved through the postures, a sense of pleasure began to flow through me, body warming up, muscles contracting and lengthening, mind quiet, breath soft. After each movement, there was rest to absorb the sensations. While in plank, I felt Chad's hand touching lightly between my shoulder blades, and he reminded me, "Soften the heart, melt the heart."

With those muscles released, a wave of energy and strength went through me, connecting the disconnected parts in me. Throughout the practice, from time to time I would feel a hand between my shoulder blades, reminding me to "melt your heart," releasing the block to the pleasant energy. Funny, this was the same message I was getting from Terry, my healer: "Listen to your heart."

Again, moving into down dog, putting the weight through my arms with my head down, I was suddenly looking into Chad's eyes. He had materialized onto the floor by my mat and was looking up at me.

"How are you doing? Does this feel ok? Is it straining your armpits?" He was looking at my scars.

"Thanks. I'm doing well."

Chad jumped up from the floor, and called out, "You rock! You just had surgery, and you are back to your yoga practice."

Confused, I didn't know whether to beam, or shrink with embarrassment.

We continued to practice, moving through series after series of postures, pausing between each to stand at the front of the mat, hands at the heart, breathing and absorbing. Instead of tiring, the energy continued to build. There was a glow that built up, an endorphin rush, like a runner's high. Continual movement for two hours.

And then, Chad said, "Come onto your backs and settle into your mats for savasana."

Ahhh, the rest portion of the yoga practice.

Lying on my back on the yoga mat in savasana with eyes closed, relaxation flowed through my limbs, trunk, head. Letting go. A warm peaceful feeling began to permeate through my body, and then began to emanate from me. A feeling of pleasant, alive warmth continued to generate from within and flow through my body structures, then beyond. Next, waves of energy started slowly coursing up through my body from my legs and pelvis out through the top of my head. Huge, intense waves, one after another, continued to move through me, building in a pleasurable, almost orgasmic way. *This must be the Kundalini!*

The waves settled into a continuous ocean of expansion until the limits of my body became blurred. Resting, I felt a calm bliss. Floating. After some time, I felt myself rising up and I was somewhere else, being hoisted up on a palette, carried at shoulder level by six people. Moving along, we entered through a cave door, dark and cool, and began to descend--down, down, down many stairs. The stairs continued down for some time, all in the darkness. When we reached the bottom step, a doorway appeared. As we moved through, the doorway opened onto a very large room, full of light. Above me was a vast expanse of sparkling ceiling. A temple! Jewels and gold decorated the ceiling and every wall. As we moved to the center of this grand place, I could see golden, jeweled pillars, beautiful statues along the walls, and several decorated altars in the center. The place was sparkling, full of light and gold everywhere. It was as if the light was golden. It seemed like a palace, but I knew it was a sacred place. Looking at the distant walls, I noticed doorways to other rooms. *This place goes on forever.* We arrived at the center of the temple and stopped by a beautiful shrine draped with a gold threaded brocade covering. As I was being moved over onto this platform, I glanced down and noticed that the floor was dirt, even though every other inch was decorated. We were deep in the earth.

A circle of people appeared out of nowhere, all dressed in golden and cream vestments, and walked forward to gather around me. *These are witnesses.* I began to feel energies shifting and moving through me, even though no one was touching me. *I am receiving a healing.* Suspended beyond time, I continued to enjoy my healing. *This is a precious experience that will enable me to know what I am to bring forward in the world.*

Eventually, the lights in this sacred place began to dim, and the energy felt more constant. As the energy was mellowing in me, I heard the sound of a bell in the distance, distinct and growing ever louder. Floating, I followed the sound with my attention, and the room around me dimmed and faded. I was again in my body, feeling my back against the yoga mat. My chest expanded with a slow, deep breath. I felt solid and radiant at the same time, aware of my entire body, even my fingers and toes. I opened my eyes and saw that the world sparkled with energy. I moved up into a cross-legged position and placed my hands in prayer at my heart. Oh, my sweet heart-- a fountain flowing from within me and bursting forth! Love. Delight danced through my whole being! I felt the hearts of everyone around me, and I knew something profound had happened here. Soul was moving freely though my body and energy system, fully enlivening me.

⁓

Soul is the vehicle of Life Force.

The soul is not simply within the body, hidden somewhere in its
    recesses.
The truth is rather the converse.
Your body is in the soul, and the soul suffuses you completely.
Therefore, all around you there is a secret and beautiful soul light.
— John O'Donahue
(Anam Cara)

At home in my meditation chair, I closed my eyes and was taken back to the first time that I had a glimpse into soul as the life force. It was decades earlier in the middle of the night while I was on call as a medical student.

"Get up! We have a Code Blue!"

A Code Blue is the term used when someone is dying and needs resuscitation. I slipped on my shoes, pulled a surgical gown on over my scrubs and scurried around the corridor trying to catch up with my resident. I rounded the corner to see a crowd of people dressed in surgical scrubs pouring out of a patient's room. Stunned. Slowing my gait, I inched up to the room. The "crash cart" with drawers flung open, was in the hallway, and a doctor (an intern?) stood in front of it, pulling medications and handing them to someone who scurried in and out of the room.

As I approached the door and peered in, I saw my fellow med student. We slipped inside against the back wall attempting to be as unobtrusive as possible. Garish! Lights were blaring. There were many beeps and whooshes and mechanical noises coming from the array of equipment that had been crowded into this room and were now attached to the patient. The patient was splayed out limp on the hospital bed, which had been moved to the center of the room, with all blankets and sheets thrown aside, her gown wadded into a wisp around her lower abdomen. There were at least ten people hovering around her, each intent and moving in a mechanical choreography, repeating the same steps over and over: watching the monitors, calling out orders, standing back, moving in. I attempted to identify the personnel: nurses, intern and resident doctors, respiratory therapist. There was a team whose job it was to respond to a Code Blue. I looked at the patient—difficult with so many people crowded around.

This woman's heart had stopped. She was immobile. I was surprised at my detachment. It didn't seem like a person at the center of this drama, but more like a machine. My mind was keen on making order out of this: calling orders, pulling open sterile packs and instruments, starting IVs and injecting drugs (one very long syringe even going through the chest and into the heart). And then there was the thrill of being included behind the scenes, allowed in rooms where there is "No Admittance".

After a while it became apparent that there was a regularity about the proceedings—a crescendo of voices and tensions as the chest compressions, injections, and then the paddles built up, and then a decrescendo when the EKG monitor began to register regular heartbeats. All eyes were drawn to the monitor and there was calm as the beep-beep-beep continued. When the beeping stopped, the attention shifted back to the patient and the routine started again. For this patient, it took an hour and a half and three rounds of resuscitation until her heart was reliably beating.

It took five people to wheel her out of the room with the attached IVs, monitors, and ventilation equipment. She was headed for the ICU. She still didn't look very alive.

Pulling back closer to the wall to let the entourage pass through the door, it struck me: after a Code Blue, the patient always leaves the room. If not to the ICU, then to the morgue.

Turning back to survey the room, it was empty except for the papers and sterile wrappers strewn on the floor. It was strangely quiet and deflated now that all the people had filed out, taking their excitement and adrenaline with them.

I was struck with what I had just witnessed: a brush with death, my first encounter in my medical training. And somehow, it didn't seem poignant or mystical, but mechanical. It seemed like trying to get an old stalled car to start and run.

There was a deep silence in the empty room...And I knew: *This patient's soul was barely inhabiting her body*—only enough to keep all her monitored functions going. Her heart was barely open. Whether she could come fully alive or not--all depended on the soul's choice to stay or go.

Opening my eyes from my memory, breathing deeply, I was moved. It occurred to me that I have had soul/body knowledge and insight throughout my life. Yet even these memories seem new. There is something more here for me to learn about how to sustain this knowing and truly access life force to integrate it into my ongoing life.

17. Out of the Cage

I HAD COME TO realize I couldn't fix my marriage.

My divorce was inevitable now.

Somehow the cage of hard thoughts around my chest had become mirrored in a larger cage that was my marriage. I had to admit that I was not thriving in the structure my marriage had become. My energy was being sapped by something that was not working, not true to my heart. Carl and I were now so far apart—but it had not always been that way.

I closed my eyes and drifted back 25 years to our honeymoon in Italy. Intimacy for newlyweds can be sweet and special, but in our case as doctors, it took on a whole other intensity.

Sitting on the outdoor deck overlooking the Mediterranean Sea at Positano, Italy, it felt as if time had stopped. We were on the final stop of our three-week honeymoon trip through Italy. It was dusk. Dinner had been perfect—every flavor fresh and savory. A warm breeze caressed us as we snuggled up together.

Carl sat up, turned and looked at me with his deep black brown eyes and said, "I want to get you pregnant!" (This from the man who was never going to have kids.)

That startled me.

"I have an IUD," I reminded him.

"We can take it out."

"OK," I said, thrilled at his snap decision.

Later that night in our hotel room, we carried out our ritual.

Pulling back the comforter on the bed, I slid off my skirt and panties and climbed in. Carl placed two pillows under my head, and I lay down and pulled my knees up to place them on the sheets by my hips. Carl sat on the side of the bed and placed his hand in my vagina, his two fingers extended toward my cervix.

"Ok. I feel the string. I think I can grasp it. Are you ready?"

There was pressure, but no pain. I could visualize exactly what he was doing.

"OK." Pressure. Pinch. He has the string now. Tug. Searing pain!

"It's not coming. I lost the string."

"It hurts. Just try again." Pinch. Pull. Pain---moving. Pressure as his hand moved out. Then relief.

"Here it is!" He held up his hand with the bloody IUD dangling from it.

"Great, "I said.

I climbed out of bed and pulled on my jeans. Carl still had the IUD draped over his finger. We started to laugh.

"Hey, let's toss it in the Mediterranean!" Carl said.

"Ooooh. Yes." I followed him out onto our deck.

Our room opened onto a balcony cut into the cliff hundreds of feet above the Mediterranean Sea. Carl walked to the edge of the guardrail and flung the IUD out into the air, aiming for the Sea far below.

The night was dark and quiet. We listened, and then burst into laughter.

"Ok, Carl. Who else in the world would find IUD removal romantic?"

He pulled me into his arms and we hugged and laughed until we stumbled onto the bed. Pulling close to each other, the world outside fell away, and we moved into a world of our own.

CRO

I smiled remembering as I opened my eyes. We did have remarkable moments.

How did we get so far apart?

I traveled to another time...

Surgeon and patient.
Shaman and dreamer.
Husband and wife.

I never could have imagined it until we were in the situation, but there was something profoundly intimate about having the man who got me pregnant operating on me when something went wrong with that pregnancy.

Five years after we were married, we were in a condo in Mexico on vacation, and in the middle of the night, our daughter Jess, came to me.

"Mommy, Mommy. I woke up. Are you ok?"

I pulled myself out of a deep sleep and looked into my three-year-old daughter's face. It was deep in the night, dark, with just a hint of moonlight from the window. The muted sound of waves and ocean breeze wafted in from the open balcony door.

"Hey, my girl. I'm ok. Did you have a bad dream?" What woke her up? She had slept soundly through the night since she was six weeks old.

"No."

Carl was sound asleep beside me. My mother in law was asleep in the large master bedroom in the back.

Raising the sheets creating a tent, I pulled my daughter into the bed with me, embracing her and planting little kisses on her neck and cheek. We snuggled up, her warm little body melding with mine. Time stopped and we were one, breathing each other in.

"Ok, Jess. We should probably get you back to bed. It's not morning yet."

Unwinding myself from the sheets, I climbed out of bed, then bending down, my arms reached to scoop her up and her arms encircled my neck. As I straightened myself up to standing, her weight transferred through my body and something snapped. Excruciating sharp pain seared through my pelvis. Immobile. Can't breathe. *OK, breathe. Don't drop Jess.* The pain radiated through my entire pelvis. Oh no! What was this?

Putting one foot in front of the other, I walked across the hall to Jess's room and lowered her into bed.

Tucking her in with a kiss, I said, "Everything is fine. You get some sleep."

I limped back to the bedroom to rouse Carl.

"Carl. Wake up! I just ruptured an ectopic."

Carl rolled over. "What?"

"I ruptured an ectopic. For sure."

"What? Are you sure? You can't do that here! We're in Mexico!"

"For sure. It broke open when I picked up Jess."

"This can't happen here. We have to get the first plane home in the morning."

"Carl, this won't wait."

"Please, Babe! Can't you do your energy thing so we can wait till tomorrow?" (He was hoping I could use some energy healing skills to delay this emergency).

"No, Too late."

Carl jumped out of bed. He got the phone number for a doctor who had retired in Puerto Vallarta and got his advice about where to get medical care.

The taxis were not working at 3:00 am, but the hospital agreed to send out an ambulance. Carl and I prepared to leave, and Jessica would stay behind with Carl's mother.

When the "ambulance" arrived, it was an open-air truck-like affair with a driver, and another man who wore an armband with a red cross on it. *He must be a medic.*

I pointed to myself and said, "Doctora." And pointed to my husband, saying "Doctor," in my best Spanish accent.

This caused the medic to start bowing to us, over and over.

"Gracias. OK. El hospital," I said.

The medic bowed, stepped aside, and Carl put a firm arm around my waist and helped me climb into the truck. In spite of the pain I felt over every bump in the road, we couldn't help but be amused.

Carl kept his arm around me and we held hands, huddled in the back of the ambulance truck. Winding down the bumpy, circuitous road, we finally reached the cobbled streets of Puerto Vallarta and pulled up in front of the CMQ hospital. We had been told that it was a private hospital, so the care should be good.

Carl and I climbed the steps of the white stucco building and went in to reception. Quickly, I was whisked to an exam room to await evaluation. Carl paced the small room, while I scanned from my seat on the exam table. *It's clean enough.* There were jars of sterile cotton balls and Q-tips on the counter, a sink, drawers and cabinets. Everything seemed to be in order. It just reminded me of how it was 20 years ago in the States.

Finally, a man came in who seemed to be the intake doctor. I desperately tried to remember my medical Spanish.

"Doctora," I started, pointing to myself.

"Embarrazada. (Pregnant). "En tubo". (In the tube.)

The doctor looked at me. "Ectopico." Hah! It's the same word in Spanish.

"Si, si."

He left the room and we waited. In a few minutes, a nurse came in and handed me a cloth gown. She opened the cabinets and pulled out a glass IV bottle and an IV needle. No plastic and Teflon here. Again 20 years ago.

We watched her every move as she placed a tourniquet on my upper arm, cleansed the skin of my forearm with Betadine on a cotton ball, wiped with a sterile gauze, and accurately inserted the needle into my bulging vein. There was a nice blood return so she inserted the tubing into the needle and started the flow of IV fluid from the glass bottle. It flowed in easily. We both breathed again. *OK, they are using sterile technique. I'm safe here.*

Carl accompanied me when they transferred me to a patient room. We realized that the attending doctor had ordered observation until morning. After a half hour just waiting, and Carl pacing, we were surprised to see a well-dressed, handsome man standing in the doorway. We had a visitor. Leandro! He had been our friend for ten years, a Columbian massage therapist and entrepreneur who worked at the Krystal Hotel. He had brought anatomy books, his fluency in Spanish, and his charisma. Both Carl and I hugged him and filled him in.

Leandro learned from the nurses that I was indeed being observed till the morning and being given IV fluids to stabilize me. Carl continued to pace around the room, more and more agitated, telling Leandro that this is viewed as much more of an emergency at home.

The pain began to worsen. Moans came from deep inside me. I heard them as if from a distance. Carl flew over to the bed and grasped the side rails, white knuckled. Tears were streaming down his face.

I touched his hand. "I'm ok. I'm going to be ok."

He was really crying now. "You are not ok! This is bad. I just wish I could operate on you."

He turned to Leandro. "Tell them she is having an emergency and needs the doctor right away!"

Leandro ran to the nurses' station.

Within 30 minutes, Dr. Lopez arrived. He was tall, gentle and soft-spoken. His English was excellent. He had trained at Guadalajara Medical School and specialized in gynecology. I was impressed that he did such a thorough physical exam, something we learn to do as med students, and then toss by the wayside in favor of technology.

"I am glad you came to this hospital, and not the public one," he said. "I have called in the radiologist and the OR staff. They are getting ready for you."

Carl was visibly relieved. He helped Dr. Lopez wheel my cart through the halls toward the radiology department. They talked about medicine in Mexico. *I think they are bonding.*

While flat on my back on the gurney, I could see only the ceiling going by. It all looked the same. Wow. I didn't like being wheeled around, not knowing where I was going. It felt vulnerable. I realized that this was what my patients experienced. It never occurred to me that just the trip through the hospital could feel so disorienting. Funny. Just the week before I was hit by the irony of how I hoped I would never have to have surgery--while at the same time I realized that my patients had to have great courage to undergo surgery when even their doctor would rather avoid it.

I was grateful that I was a gynecologist and knew what was going on. I shuddered to think what might happen to a patient of mine in a foreign country. A patient in my situation probably wouldn't know how serious this could be. They could die. I could have died.

Carl squeezed my hand as we walked through the halls.

When we arrived at our destination we met another doctor—another tall, handsome doctor. He had a new ultrasound machine that he proudly showed to Carl.

The three doctors (Carl, Lopez, and Perez) moved me onto the exam table. In order to use the ultrasound, I needed a full bladder, so the nurses had been pouring IV fluids into me and I had not urinated. My full bladder pushed on the pelvic structures causing more pain, but it helped the doctor to see on the ultrasound.

Dr. Perez had positioned the screen so we could all see as he scanned. The cool gel on the ultrasound wand touched my skin.

Ugh. Even that small amount of pressure caused increased pain. He maneuvered the wand and pulled a good picture into view on the screen. "Ohhh", we all murmured in recognition. It was a definite ectopic.

"Wow. That is excellent resolution." Carl complimented Dr. Perez and his new ultrasound machine, as he stepped closer to the screen to look.

"Well, look at this." Soon I could no longer see the ultrasound screen as three doctor heads crowded out my view. They were appreciating this wonderful new equipment and trying out all the features. Boys and their toys.

"You guys, I'm in pain here. I need to empty my bladder. Can you operate on me now?"

The three doctors started and turned to look at me.

"Sorry, Mar. This is just such a great piece of equipment," Carl said, and he returned to my side.

We left Dr. Perez with his ultrasound machine and wheeled me upstairs. We passed through a set of double doors and I was parked (on my gurney) in an anteroom. Another set of double doors on the opposite side of the anteroom stood wide opening into the operating room. The operating table stood at the center, and a woman in sterile gown, gloves, hat and mask worked busily to prepare for surgery. The room looked familiar with the large lights over the table, the sterile drapes and packs waiting to be opened, an anesthesia machine by the head of the table.

Dr. Lopez spoke to the woman in Spanish, then turned to me and said, "This is Guadalupe, the scrub nurse. She will be here with you while we prepare for surgery."

"Can she put the Foley in now?" I was miserable with the extra pressure in my bladder and wanted to have it emptied with a catheter.

"Yes, of course. Carl and I will go for coffee while we wait for you to be prepared."

"Ok, Mar? We will be close by," Carl said, and kissed me.

"Sure."

Dr. Lopez and Carl left, and the nurse Guadalupe came to me to place a Foley catheter in my bladder. Ahhhh, relief. As the bladder was drained, the pressure in my pelvis was relieved and the pain decreased to its dull constant baseline. *Better.*

Guadalupe spoke to me in Spanish, and although I didn't understand all her words, I could tell from her tone that she was reassuring me. I gleaned that this was a good hospital, the doctors were excellent, some American women came here to get their face-lifts from the famous plastic surgeon who was on staff here. Guadalupe didn't want me to worry. I was not worried, now that I knew I would have surgery.

Bang! The double doors burst open to reveal a tall, dark attractive man dressed in tight-fitting jeans, cowboy boots, and a T-shirt that said, "Party Animal". He strode over to my gurney, lifted the designer shades from his eyes and leaned over me to peer at my face.

"Anestesiólogo," Guadalupe called from the operating room.

Whoa! This is my anesthesiologist?

He nodded, and then moved to the opposite wall. It was then that I noticed this room was lined with hooks, some which had clothes hanging on them. The anesthesiologist started taking his clothes off down to his underwear, and then put on surgical scrubs before walking into the OR! No locker rooms in this Mexican hospital. The pre-op holding area doubled as the changing room.

After a while, Carl and Dr. Lopez returned.

Carl walked over to me, grabbed my hand, and leaned down to whisper in my ear, "I'm going to do your surgery. Ricardo only does three or four ectopics a year."

Tears welling up for us both. He kissed my forehead.

"Oh, good. I'm glad they will let you do it."

"Yeah. They don't have laparoscopy here, so it is the old open laparotomy technique, but I'll do a tiny incision."

We shared relief.

I was then wheeled into the OR while Carl and Dr. Lopez changed into scrubs.

The anesthesiologist moved me onto my side and started to prep my back with Betadine.

"Are you giving me a spinal?" I asked.

"Epidural."

Wow. That's advanced! I would be awake for my surgery! YAY! I could talk to Carl blow by blow.

Once the epidural tube was positioned into the space above the spine, and taped into place, I was repositioned on my back, and draped for surgery. As the medication started to seep in, the pain slowly dulled and disappeared. Carl and Dr. Lopez scrubbed and came into the OR to receive sterile towels for drying their hands. Next, they were dressed with sterile gowns and gloves—a comforting and universal routine.

"Carl, I have an epidural! We will be able to talk during the procedure!" I said.

"Great, Babe! I will tell you everything."

Carl took his place to my right in the surgeon's position, Dr. Lopez at my left in the assistant surgeon's position, Guadalupe on the other side of Dr. Lopez, facing Carl, and the anesthesiologist at my head, out of my view.

"Ready?" Carl asked the anesthesiologist. When he got the nod, he held his hand out to Guadalupe. "Scalpel."

Carl and I had operated together so many times through the past ten years, beginning with our residency, taking turns being the primary surgeon or the assistant. We moved as one, anticipating each next step without having to speak. There was an intimate zone that we would step into together—shaman surgeons for the patient. The surgeries were so smooth together, we set records for time: we could often do a C-section or a hysterectomy in 25 minutes. We had a reputation among the hospital staff for efficiency, time, and good outcomes. "Bloodless surgery." We worked in the healing zone.

Surgeons and patient
    Shamans and dreamer...

Because of our experience together in the OR, I could picture exactly what Carl was doing even though I couldn't see the surgical field. Dr. Lopez translated so Guadalupe knew what instruments to pass to Carl.

I began to feel sleepy. Wait! "Are you putting me to sleep?" I asked the anesthesiologist.

"No. It's Valium," he said. This guy was not a talker. It wasn't because he didn't understand me. I felt so out of control.

"Please don't. I want to know what's going on. Is there any way I can watch?"

"No, Mar. I don't think you can watch. We have to keep you draped," Carl said. "I'm down to the fascia."

"Ok." My attention focused on the fascia and all the steps to open the abdomen, and then I was in the zone with Carl.

I am the patient/dreamer.

He is the surgeon/shaman.

"I'm just getting in the peritoneum. Wow—it's ruptured all right. Suction!"

"There is no suction machine," Dr. Lopez said.

Carl sopped up the blood with laparotomy sponges. I could see it in my mind's eye, and feel his hands somehow on a different level, cleaning up, and no pain.

"The tube is really blown. I can't save it," Carl said to me.

"That's ok, Babe. Do the right thing."

Carl deftly dissected the tube away from its attachments and handed it off to the circulating nurse.

"Irrigation," Carl called.

A minute later he said, "Mar, they gave me the water in a pitcher. I don't know if I should pour it in. I hope it's sterile—we don't even drink the water here!" (In the OR in the US, the sterile water comes in plastic sterilized bottles.)

"I'm sure it's fine." We had a good laugh, and he proceeded to rinse my peritoneal cavity, sopping up the bloody fluid with dry laparotomy sponges.

A few minutes later, the circulating nurse brought the specimen over to show me. That really touched me. It was a bloody fallopian tube sitting in the middle of a green surgical towel, splayed open with clot and conceptus spilling out. Nothing identifiable as an embryo yet. I felt Carl pause as I inspected the little pregnancy gone astray.

"Sorry baby. Still no home for you. We will get you here somehow," I whispered. I felt Carl and knew even as he was operating, there were tears in his eyes. This was the third pregnancy loss we had had since Jessica was born—the other two were miscarriages—and we were at a loss, together.

Carl finished closing the incision, helped remove the drapes, and came over to me. He took my hand from under the drape, bent down, and kissed my cheek, letting go of the role of surgeon and relaxing into being my husband. He whispered, "We'll try again."

I was transferred to a hospital room and instantly fell into a deep sleep.

Later that evening, I sat up in my hospital bed, moved into a cross-legged position, and breathed easily. There was no pain at all, and no need for pain meds. Nice! I closed my eyes and drifted into a meditative state. A wave of gratitude moved through me for the opportunity to share this surgery with Carl. Another feeling came over me, and I knew it was the presence of the little soul trying to come as our child. This was the same one that had been trying to come all along. We hadn't lost anyone. Calm. Peace. All is well. *Thank you for being near. We will find a way for you to come.*

It had been a true healing, with Carl being the surgeon healer, and also my husband. I had been his patient, his surgical buddy and his wife and had accepted the healing.

Surgeon and patient.
Shaman and dreamer.
Husband and wife.
Parents...

What had happened to us? We had a reliable connection to spirit as surgeons healing together and as parents. Together, we had created something of value in this world. In these areas we were in tune, close, expanded, inspired. We complemented each other.

But then something changed. When we grew larger as a practice, and stopped doing surgery together, we even lost that source of intimacy. As the years passed, our practice together grew and became more successful, but we were no longer connecting. He was the business master behind it all. In the beginning, it was exhilarating to support him. He achieved his mission of a multi-location full service women's practice that was the premiere practice in the Northwest suburbs of Chicago. When we started, we put our heads together, but as time went on, I felt more and more invisible to Carl. I was only on his radar if I complained that I was tired and wanted to work less, and then he was tyrannous, to pressure me to keep the system going. He counted on me to continue my productive practice that attracted so many patients, but he became too busy to have a personal relationship with me. Mutuality eluded us.

Now, it was finally time to admit to myself that we were not going to come back together. He had strayed too far. Staying in this trap for so long had made me tired, weary, invisible even to myself. My work all day was helping women regain their health by opening to their soul's truth. It was time for me. I had entered the cage willingly, and it was now time to set myself free. Still, it was a big step. It felt like the right decision, but how could I know?

One dusky evening, pondering my decision, I drove down the lane to my home, and something caught my eye in the trees above me. *A bird. An owl.* A sense of peace flooded me. I smiled as I remembered another big moment in my life when an owl had been present for another difficult decision. It was a when I had decided to give up being an Obstetrician to be a Gynecologist only.

It was Dec 30, 2000, and I was driving home from delivering my last baby. Having decided to retire from OB, I was looking forward to more time with my daughters. I was surprised at the rush of emotions that poured out after I did the delivery.

Snow flurried over the windshield. It was dusk, that eerie cusp between light and dark. During the winding drive up Northwest Highway, tears came and went. *Did I make the right decision? I am a good obstetrician. Maybe I will go back to it when my girls are grown...*

I turned onto the lane that led to my driveway. Still snowing and starting to get dark, then whoosh—*what was that? An enormous bird swooped down and started flying ahead of me down the road. What is this? Wingspan must be 6 feet. Is it a hawk? Can't tell.* Driving slowly down the lane, the bird was leading.

Nearing the end of the road, just as it seemed the bird was about to fly off, he continued ahead, suddenly swooping up and perching on a tree that arched over my driveway. He seemed to be waiting for me. I pulled into the driveway and looked up. A large owl, three feet tall, majestic and wise, stared down at me. His presence was magical. He was witness somehow to my journey.

A sense of peace descended—Ahhhh. *This owl has put a blessing on my decision, my homecoming.* Another glimmer from the other world. More tears, this time tears of wonder and relief. All is well.

Continuing up the long, winding driveway, then into the garage. I walked into the mudroom and called out, "Everybody come! Hello! I have something amazing to tell you!" Quiet. I pulled off my coat, walked to the kitchen, picked up the phone and pushed the intercom..."Where are you? Come now."

"We're watching a movie," Jess answered.

"Pause it. I have something amazing to tell you."

"OK."

Carl pulled himself away from the computer.

Finally, the family was assembled in the kitchen and I told them of my owl guide.

Thirteen-year-old eyes stared at me and calculated, absorbed. No comment. Olivia, age 8, eyed her sister, then me, then said, "Cool, Mom. Can we finish the movie?"

According to Greek mythology, an owl sat on Athena's blind side, so that she could see the whole truth. Often myth indicates the owl accompanying a spirit to the underworld winging its newly freed soul from the physical world into the realm of spirit. That night, lying in bed, I remembered: In mythology, the owl is seer of souls, the keeper of spirits who pass from one plane to another. The owl is considered a symbol of wisdom and truth. Rather than intellectual wisdom, though, owls are connected with the wisdom of the soul.

I had been blessed, visited by a spirit guide to usher me into a new phase of my life. Seeing this owl, I relaxed. I was again at the threshold of another phase in my life and had received a nod from spirit. *The decision to divorce is right for me now*

The next day I arose the and composed an email to my dearest friends. It was a call for connection, prefaced with an apology for being out of touch and consumed with getting back to my own truths.

"I consider each of you as someone whom I have connected with and trusted--even if it has been some time since we have been in contact.

"I am at a transition point in my life, and I realize I need connection and support from friends. When under pressure/ stress, I tend to withdraw and I feel somewhat like I have lived under a rock for the past several decades. I am going through a divorce and I have had many realizations about myself as I go through this difficult but necessary process.

"I have been remembering myself before this marriage, and how I loved my work and always had validation and support around me--I felt valued and seen at work and in my personal relationships. But for the past 20 years my work and home environment have become unhealthy--where I was suspected, betrayed, kept off balance, and I have become weird and tenta- tive. I realize that this is because I have not lived in Truth with myself. I missed all the opportunities along the way to say— 'this is wrong for me,' and I have pretended that we are ok, while behind the scenes I have been miserable."

We'd been on a treadmill to make money, my intimate part- nership had vanished a long time ago, my partner had even be- trayed me, and we were just pretending in public. I had become physically exhausted and unhealthy.

It was hard, being a doctor, telling others of my vulnerability, but this letter was important.

"I realize that I have done good work and have been blessed to bring in integrated knowledge from Source/God. I have won- derful relationships with my daughters. And there is more to come from me.

"But somehow over the last 25+ years, I have lived without 'my people' at work and at home (or have not been fully able to receive those around me). I have been spooked and inauthentic...not living in my Truth. Next weekend we will tell our girls about our plans for divorce--and to me this marks the time of being able to speak truthfully... (If you are close by--please wait till after June 5th to speak of this...)

"I am ready to come home to myself and be a good and connected friend. I commit to you all that I will show up, be in truth, and be authentic.

"Please, if the Spirit moves you, connect with me. I can be a tough/shy cookie.

"Several of you have been great to keep connecting with me. I am grateful beyond words...

"So--please think of me, pray for me, ask me out, visit me, email me, make plans with me---I need to rebuild my strong net of connection.

"If you made it through this long email, thank you. Would love to hear from you.

"Love and hugs and blessings, Marilyn"

18. The Angel of Cancer

I WAS BEGINNING TO feel a whole new sense of relaxation in my being. Smiling for no reason. Feeling the delight. I felt myself trusting and expecting the guidance I was getting in my meditations and healings.

One morning when I sat down to meditate, I asked myself:

What do I want?
What is the longing?
And my heart answered:
Oh! To wake up every morning with delight to start a new day.
    Carry a delighted heart and radiant self throughout the day.
        Pure ecstasy in all I do.
            Ecstasy. Radiance.
Surrender the cage and rigid posture of habit.
    Habitual tension.
Trust the Love to well up from the River of life.
    Soothing all the little holdout places
        Pouring in from all sides
            Carried by pure Light through my day
Open the spaciousness.

Smiling, I recalled a discussion with Terry after a recent healing. He had asked me, "When was the last time you did a healing on yourself, where you actually put yourself on the table and went through all the steps?"

Well, it had been years. What was my resistance?

"It would be a good thing for you to do at this point in your healing journey," Terry had said.

As a healer, I knew it was possible to access a holographic representation of one's own body on the healing table and then work on healing oneself through the hologram.

I struggled with feelings of reluctance but resolved to make time for this healing. I had no idea how profound the experience would be.

I chose a time when I could be alone in my room. The healing table was in the center of the room, prepared with a pillow, sheets and my favorite native blanket. I took a step back from the table and planted my feet, sending energy roots down into the earth for grounding. My arms at my sides slowly reached out and arced above my head, reaching to the heavens. The flow of energy coursed through me, joining heaven and earth, and circulated through me, waking up all my chakras, meridians, organs, cells, senses.

Reaching up with open palms, I felt the energy form of my body, the hologram, drifting into my grasp. As if holding a baby, I guided this form down to the healing table, then ran my hands over the hologram to feel the dimensions. As my hands touched the energy that was my hologram form, it became visible to me: shimmery, glistening light. Some healers see energy directly, but I feel it kinesthetically first, and this allows me to see it. I ran my fingers over my scalp, head face, then moved to my chest, arms, trunk, and legs until the entire form was clearly outlined. The organs became visible within the form—the liver, kidneys, bowels. Wherever my hands touched, structures became clear.

I moved to the foot of the healing table, raised my hands and began to move them in a rhythm to clear the auric levels and grid structures. Next, I moved back to the side of the table and beginning at the first chakra, I sensed the vortex of energy and cleared and reinforced its structure with my two hands. I continued working on each chakra.

As I worked, I gradually became aware of a presence standing on the other side of the table. Looking up, I saw the form of a woman. I was awestruck by her beauty. She moved close to the table. She was exactly my size, standing across from me and mirroring me. This was no ordinary person, she was fearsomely beautiful with shining thick hair cascading to her waist. Her features and her form were slightly blurred by the light that emanated from within her and extended from all around her. We looked at one another. Her eyes shone and bore into mine. We were silently sharing, energy flowing between us, merging and melding. I realized this extraordinary vision was the Angel of Cancer. How ironic! I never expected her to be so beautiful.

From the upper corner of the field, a glistening crystal began to slowly descend toward me. As it came closer, I realized that it was an energetic geode, cracked open. The outside was a half sphere with a rough surface and the inside was bursting with white crystal, rose quartz, and amethyst, growing from within and shining out. It was exquisite.

Continuing its descent, the crystal seated itself into the chest area of my energy body on the table. A warm glow rose up in me from this vibrant new source of energy.

This dazzling object, this crystal, was a gift to me from her. The amazing crystalline structure was beauty and promise, and its inner beauty carried a special vibration for me.

Out of a seemingly dark mass, an unexpected gem.

Just like the cancer mass—deep within there was an unexpected beauty.

I was no longer afraid. No longer tentative. I was captivated and ready to face the Angel of Cancer. Waves of energy pulsed through me. The cage structure that had surrounded my heart was beginning to soften and become more flexible.

As I stood at the healing table, energy both poured into me and flowed out. Beams of warm light flowed into my heart center from the heavens, from the beautiful spirit, and from my energy body on the table, lighting up my whole being. And then, my heart center swelled and the light poured forth from me, connecting again with my energy body, and flowing to the spirit to complete the circuit, and then from my heart out into the world.

My experience could be a healing message to others. I heard:
There is an unlimited supply of love energy.
I am power. I am light. I am timeless.

The healing was slowly coming to an end.
I looked deeply at this being, taking her in fully, and said:

Thank you for this incredible gift. You are a beautiful being and teacher. You took me below the surface and opened me to myself. I have heard you and seen you. I accept the gift you have brought me and I will remember always.
I am ready to release you now and be healed.

She nodded, bowed deeply, stepped back and then was gone.
My new heart, new power, and new life remained.

After my encounter with the Angel of Cancer, I began to feel more confident in reconnecting to my own spirit on a deep level. There was something very comforting about knowing that I had given the cancer my thoughtful attention. Facing cancer and its meaning for me was allowing me to feel my personal power.

Afterward, I sat in my meditation chair and a wave of gratitude moved through me. *How blessed I am to be able to connect with the spirit world!* Closing my eyes, I went back to another time eighteen years earlier when I learned how to open and access information from the spirit world with my newborn second daughter Olivia:

Standing in the family room of our small temporary home, with my three-week old baby secure in my arms, I sighed with contentment. Fatigue washed through my body, making even my brain slow. The radiant warmth of this new infant was the only energy motivating me to move. We were still one being—just split into two interconnected units. Her heart was so wide open that my heart opened too. I stopped and absorbed her energy, swaying and rocking her, looking into her bright eyes. As we flowed our energy freely with each other, my body limits began to blur. I hugged her close, and after some time I realized I was seeing through her perspective! In this deeply relaxed and open state, I was able to access information from my baby. She was an amazingly calm baby and was sharing information with me, transmitting a wealth of knowledge, and my mind was rapidly translating it into words:

"I have lived many times before and am happy to be here again. It is difficult for a soul to be contained in a small body— many are uncomfortable and cry since there is so little control. We babies are helpless, picked up, clothes changed, put to bed, moved around. I just ride with it, rock with it. The time was right for me to come."

I was actually feeling everything from her perspective first— and then my mind was describing it. It was delicious. Another part of my mind was stunned. This was an answer to the question I posed when I was pregnant: What is it like for little souls to come into their bodies? And now, through my newborn, I was receiving an answer—a look into her world of beginning life.

As the information continued to flow in, I was surprised at how open I was, and deeply moved. I was in such an open state of being that I had made a direct spirit connection and was able to receive her transmissions.

I settled into my overstuffed chair with her in my arms and continued the experience. All was right with the world.

These transmissions continued through the first year of Olivia's life. One time when she was eight months old I was standing in the kitchen ready to walk out the door for work. Looking back at my baby sitting on the kitchen floor, I felt a pang about leaving her again. My mind softened, her brown eyes held mine, and I heard: Don't worry. I have a whole life going on when you are gone. I have my nanny and my sister and I am happy. You don't take my life when you go away. And I am still here for you when you return.

In this way, I would access helpful information from her when I had questions that concerned her.

The transmissions were a wonderful reminder that we are all souls who emerge from the spirit world and come into our human bodies. When we are born, we are still connected to our vast souls, but we lose that conscious connection as we begin organizing our lives with our linear minds. How profound that I had found a portal to that spirit world once again!

As Olivia developed language, this type of telepathy slowed down, and it became rare that for me to receive transmissions from her directly into my thoughts. However, she has had a life of predictive dreams, premonitions, and sensitivity to psychic information.

As I reflected on this early time with Olivia, a thrill of recognition ran through me. This time was when I first opened the door to access helpful information directly from a person's spirit/soul. After that I was able to do this with my patients. I was stunned by how profoundly helpful this unique ability was. It could guide me to a patient's deeper concerns, underlying and undetected disease, and best treatment approaches. I was able to listen to their deeper truth and help them to free themselves from their own thought cages.

I regularly used this access with my patients, but it hadn't occurred to me to use it for myself. Why is it so easy to see what others need and how to help them heal, but so difficult to recognize these needs in myself? It was clear that my cage of habitual thoughts had kept me in the role of doctor and helper, somehow aloof and blind to the cage itself. I had been the observer and facilitator for others to move toward healing while holding myself removed from my own heart's truth and my own healing.

Sitting in my meditation chair and remembering the Angel of Cancer and the many patients whose spirits had spoken to me, I felt a growing desire within me to connect and never let go—to find a way to truly live in connection. I closed my eyes and heard:

You have discovered the keys, They are three:

First, open the gate (the cage: outmoded thoughts and habits).

Second, your heart will then naturally flow with spirit, connecting to your soul.

Third, find your voice.

You have known this and it is unfolding for you.

As I heard these words, I felt a great sense of peace. I saw a bird emerging from her cage, stretching and opening her wings, then flying free with strength, grace, and ease. After some time, she glided to a landing on a high perch and began to sing.

She is a dove, and carries feminine energies, peace, and prophecy.

I am a dove, like my father.

Opening my eyes, I smiled. All is well.

19. Flying Free

I COULD FEEL MY freedom just around the corner.

Summer was drawing to a close. The car was packed with all of Olivia's belongings, and we would soon be heading cross-country to Massachusetts where she would start her first year at Mount Holyoke College.

My children are launched. Freedom.

Carl and I were nearly finished with the divorce settlement we designed together. Despite many disagreements, there was a sweet calm and poignancy between us as we worked out the final details. When we told our daughters (now 18 and 23) that we were getting a divorce, they weren't surprised. We had decided to continue all our family traditions, and Carl would keep the house, so I would be moving.

My difficult marriage was ending. Freedom.

Leaving home. Freedom.

A week earlier, my yoga intensive immersion sessions ended. The day before our final closure, Chad again led us through another long and energizing yoga practice. Usually, it would have seemed impossible to move continually for over two hours through one strenuous and contorted pose sequence after another, but the longer we continued, the more energized I felt. My continually renewing energy was more than just improved circulation or an endorphin rush. It was as if energy from an outside source was finding its way into my body and enlivening it. Chad recited the formula for this: "Set the Foundation. Open to Grace. Engage muscular energy. Now Shine Out!" It worked in building waves of energy and bliss.

Finally, he brought the asana practice to a close. As we settled onto the mat for savasana, my body began to tingle with anticipation. Again, the kundalini waves of energy began to move through me, and I felt an expansion, and then again hanging in a floating state of bliss. After some time, I felt myself being carried on a palette, but this time the path was upward. Up and up through clouds to the heavens on what felt like endless white stairs. After what felt like some time, I arrived at a door. I was carried through the doorway, across a threshold and into a vast sacred temple, which was entirely white with gold trim at the base of the pillars, around the arches. Again, I was placed on a platform for healing, which was draped in a richly decorated all white quilt. As before, a circle of witnesses again gathered around me. Everyone was dressed in white gowns. My healing proceeded with energies moving and shifting through me in an indescribably precious and palpable way. It was heavenly. When I emerged from this healing back onto my yoga mat, I was again changed. Not only did I receive a healing, but I was anointed as a healer: shown the profound healing power of connecting soul into the body.

Connecting with the soul connects one to God (Spirit).
Soul is the vehicle of Life Force.

The practice of yoga had initiated a profound experience--integrating an upgrade to my mind body, spirit, and preparing and strengthening me for my independence. My body was thinner and stronger than it had been in years.

Strong, healthy body. Freedom.

My radiation therapy with healing sessions completed the same week—six weeks, five days per week. No more treatments were required. On the last day after my final treatment, the technician walked over to move the canisters and help me sit up. As I sat on the side of the treatment table and pulled the earbuds out of my ears, I noticed three other staff members walking across the room to me. The four women formed a semi-circle around me and spoke:

"We are sorry you had cancer, but very happy to have been able to meet you."

"It was always a pleasure to have you come in."

"You made the whole center peaceful."

"I felt like I got the healing on the mornings you were here."

"You have grace and peace around you."

"Please come back and tell us more about the healing, now that you are no longer a patient."

Tears rimmed my eyes. Surprise. I had no idea that I could have that much impact. I heard the words, *Your healing will benefit many.*

Completion of cancer treatment—Freedom.

It seemed that all the threads of my life were converging to support me in my step to freedom. There was a new skip in my step. Delight for no reason. All that remained was to take Olivia to college and then find a new home for myself.

As we pulled around on our driveway to start the journey to college, we stopped by our coach house where my mom lived. Olivia jumped out of the car to meet Mom as she came from her house and walked around the car. Last goodbyes.

"Goodbye Gram! I will be back at Thanksgiving."

"Have a great start, Honey. Be careful. I miss you already." Then coming to the driver's door, she leaned in and kissed my cheek. "Be careful driving, Honey." She was holding back the tears.

We drove on around the curve of the driveway, and as we neared the end, a dove glided by in front of us. Olivia and I looked at each other and smiled. *Grandpa.*

Arriving back home from my trip to take Olivia to college, I felt my excitement building. Soon I would be free of the entanglements that had been tying me down. *Freedom.* There was also the matter of finding a place to live. Within a few weeks, our divorce would be final, and I would need to move. One moment I was feeling anxiety and pressure, and the next moment I was dancing with elated anticipation. It was as if my mind and heart were vying for the driver's seat.

My emotions were high—all of them. Was it ecstasy or anxiety? It seemed that I vacillated between the two or felt both simultaneously. Whatever it was, I was more alive than I had been in a long time.

Soon after my return was the appointment for my first follow up mammogram after treatment. Walking into the reception area, I noticed the beautiful earth tone Zen decor of the Breast Center but somehow it seemed all wrong. Usually, this would have made me feel peaceful, but today it was annoying to me. *What is wrong with me?* As I walked back with the technician for the testing, it hit me. The last time I was here, they found more cancer than expected. *I am nervous. No... scared.* Although my external demeanor was as calm as always, I was shaking inside. *I hate being vulnerable.* As a healer, I knew that the body often holds memories in the cells, and this was why my body was reacting. I understood, but I was still annoyed.

Soon I was distracted by having to maneuver my breasts onto the mammogram plates and then feeling the squeeze of the machine. Then repeat on the other side...

Afterward I dressed hurriedly and rushed out of the building. Safely in my car, I did my yoga breathing and moved on. *It has to be fine.*

A few hours after the mammogram was taken, my cell phone rang. I had just pulled into the grocery parking lot. I picked up my phone and the words "Breast Center" lit up the screen. Yikes. *Why do I have to answer?*

It was Leslie, director of the Breast Center, who hurried to tell me, "I got the radiologist to read your mammogram as soon as he arrived. It is negative. No cancer detected. Really good news, Marilyn."

"Thank you, Leslie. You are the best."

I am cancer free. I hung up the phone, sat in my car, and sobbed.

I was feeling more alive than ever, radiant, hopeful. I was ready to be free and have a beautiful perfect home of my own.

But, something was off. My realtor and friend Kathy had shown me dozens of homes, but nothing really felt right to me. Doubt started to creep in.

Why couldn't I find my home? I questioned in my journal. The cage door had been opening, the rigid bars softening, and I was more peaceful and happy. In my meditation and healing, I saw the cage transforming and my outer life had begun to reflect an inner shift. I had done my inner work. Why wasn't my home manifesting before me?

I closed my eyes and began to breathe deeply. As I relaxed and settled, I again saw the cage, more ephemeral than before. It seemed to be pulsing, at times more defined, and then more faded. As I observed it, something remarkable happened: it faded, and then unwound until it was reorganized into an open structure. It felt like home. *A home, not a prison.* And then it came more clearly into focus and I saw that it was actually a nest. The thoughts and beliefs were more flexible and supportive. I basked in this support for a while, knowing that I had grown and opened. And then after a time, I saw the cage again. It became clear and prominent. The nest had not disappeared but had faded somewhat. I knew this was a reminder that I might slip back into the limited thinking of the cage at times, but it was a choice.

I saw this phenomenon in my patients, but now I understood it from the inside. Remarkable.

I opened my eyes and smiled.

⁓

That night, I decided to look on the internet for my house. I clicked through thirty listings and found two that I was willing to see. And then I clicked on a house that sent a charge through me. I said aloud, "That's what I'm talking about!"

The next day, Kathy brought me to the houses I had asked to see. We pulled up to the special house that I had chosen on line. Nestled in a neighborhood in the village of Barrington, the stucco house and neat yard looked inviting. Walking up the sidewalk to the porch steps, I felt a wonderful thrill of delight. I walked up the steps to the porch. *I could sit here in the evening.* Kathy unlocked the door and swung it open.

Stepping across the threshold onto the warm honey-colored hardwood floor, I caught my breath. I walked into the small foyer and scanned the space. A sense of peace surrounded me as the sunlight streamed through the beveled glass windows and warmed me. My eyes scanned the open living room/dining room expanse and found original woodwork with built-in cabinetry from 1913. There was even an elaborate woodworked ceiling. The energy was scintillating and palpable. I was swimming in peace and delight. *This feels like home.*

Walking through the rest of the house, I rounded the corner on the second floor and walked into a small room. *My meditation and yoga room.* Another room—*My office.* At the end of the hall—*my bedroom.*

As I walked back down the crafted staircase, and stood again in the front entryway, I knew I could live here. Kathy took me to look at several other houses, and sometimes while I was away I would doubt my first experience in the stucco house, but whenever I would step back into the house, I would have that same feeling: *This feels like home.*

The last time I went to look at the house before I decided to buy it, I looked out the window and saw a cardinal sitting in the tree in the front yard. Confirmation.

When I bought my house, I knew that I was that bird, the dove, from my meditation, released from her cage who had found her perfect safe place. Home.

> the birds have flown to freedom
> the cage lies empty
> your happy songs bring me the scent of heaven
> please keep singing!
> —Rumi

Bird
  Being.
  Breathing.
    Bringing in my Higher Self.
Having my wits about me but being out of my mind.
Delight creeping in—
    Singing my song.
I am the songbird
    The Lark
    The Dove
    The Phoenix
Flying free—living with delight.

Loosening the grip of hard thoughts
For love to flow in and give my heart wings.

༄

Birds had always been a part of my life, but now I seemed to see them everywhere. They surrounded me to encourage me, inspire me, remind me that there was a world beyond the mundane. They demonstrated how to fly strong and free, how to nest, how to sing. I felt like one of them, a bird freed from her cage learning to be wild, spirited and free.

Often, the cardinal and white dove would appear, and I would feel the presence of Aunt Bettie and my father. But as the months progressed, I began to see hawks, an eagle, egrets, hummingbirds, and sweet robins. For a time, every morning half a dozen blue jays sat in a tree as I was driving off to work, squawking and hollering at me. It seemed they were urging me to speak up—find my voice.

It became apparent that the birds were Couriers of Spirit and appeared at times in my life when big change was happening.

It was an exhilarating time, but there were still some parts of my life that required healing.

20. Connecting with Divine Feminine

My cancer was gone.
I had my perfect new home.
I was free.
So, what was missing?

NOW THAT I WAS in a cozy, peaceful home that felt safe and warm, I was reconnecting with friends, going out. There was more laughter. Fun. I felt attractive again. My friends even commented on the difference. Younger. Bright. Happy. I felt delighted!

But then there were the other times. Coming in after a wonderful evening with friends to an empty house. Driving home from work at the end of the day. Alone.

One evening, I came into my house, tossed my keys on the counter, and threw my coat on the couch. The sad feeling came over me again. *Alone.* Dragging myself to my meditation room, I sank into the chair. Why is this happening? Silence. Dense silence. After a time, I felt something let go inside of me, releasing my hold on my frustration. I closed my eyes and breathed more deeply. *Ok, I'm listening. What do I need to know?*

Slowly a feeling of gentleness came over me. The tight ball of sadness seemed to gradually expand so that it was lighter.

Movement. Flow. Gentle waves. As I relaxed, I noticed that my soul energy was infusing the ball of sadness and allowing it to move, to not be alone. This sad aloneness was one of the oldest emotions I had buried within. A holdout. Even though I had softened my inner cage, and set myself free in the world, the old pattern wasn't completely healed.

Breathing. Letting go. Peace flowed through me and the flow of Source through me became stronger, consistent, until all the traces of the tight ball were carried away on the river. I am not alone. Peace. Quiet.

As I indulged in the quiet, I heard myself ask, *What do I need to hear?*

Silence. And then I heard:

The cage of hard thoughts was formed when you were very young, and got stronger through the years. There were people in your life that did not see or hear you, who hurt you, who abandoned you. This is unfortunate, but they are not to blame for your cage. They have limitations and their own illusions and suffering. The cage was formed when you did not listen to your own voice, when you abandoned yourself. Putting the blame on another pulled your attention outside yourself, and you fashioned your own cage when you were cut off from the truth in your heart, and cut off from your soul connection.

You have freed yourself from the cage that binds you. Now it is time to call your attention back to your own heart. Do not abandon yourself.

This was a deeper level of truth with myself...

As I meditated, these words came:

Communicate Love
Ah, I am vast—
   I had forgotten...

I am capable of connecting
   With Love
      Source
        Flow
Even when you feel cut off
   And afraid
      And feel like you're falling
        Into the dark.
Extend vast Love flow

I can feel only this
Communicate only this

Nothing can separate me from the love of God.
As I sat, a feeling of overwhelming peace began to grow from within. Grace descending. I was plugged in to a flow that supported me. Source River.
I can feel this no matter where I am.

Grace descend
   Be with me
Flow through my body
   Open my love and peace
Flow through my head, eyes, jaw
   Through my sadness
      Aloneness
Burst up through my heart like a fountain.
Peace in the land—
   In the terrain of my body
Even in the midst of upset others
Be the River that flows around the stressed ones
   bringing soothing water
      to their island shores.
Being peace, flow, love.

A more consistent peace began to permeate my life. When I felt emotions rising I would more often remember to stop and listen to my inner truth. Listening to my inner truth took practice and patience. After each round of connecting, and a peaceful interval, another wave of emotion would rise. Gradually, I was forging an ever-deepening access to my authentic self. The tricky part for me was acknowledging my emotions. My habit of attempting to solve everything by using my mind made it difficult to even realize I was having deep emotions, they had been so effectively walled off by my mind. I began to see how my pattern of putting the linear mind in charge of quelling or ignoring emotions was a way of reverting to the caged approach to life.

One morning I sat in my meditation chair, closed my eyes, and breathed deeply. How can I have this peacefulness more easily? After some time, I heard these words:

Mind takes charge
So the messiness of emotion
 Can be stuffed in the closet
  Quelled
  Quieted.
And the hum of regular, neat life can march cleanly. Perfect.

But then something gnaws a little
 A headache
  A feeling
   A sadness
    A hollowness in the chest
Cut off—alone.

And the mind tenses
 Hardens

Becomes frantic
Adamant.
Stuck.

Until the feeling, the headache, the sadness
Begins to trickle,
Open
Release
Flow.
Pouring, flooding

And finally, then even the mind softens
Takes notice
Makes space.

Mind and Heart
Masculine and Feminine
Yang and Yin
Coming together to make peace in the Land.

Opening my eyes, I smiled, liking the idea of Mind and Heart making peace in the Land. My mind had been the authority— the Masculine Principle. My heart had been curtailed—the Feminine Principle. And Heart is the connection to the Divine Feminine! Although I had made much progress in opening and listening to my heart, I had not fully connected with the spirit of the divine feminine.

A sense of longing expanded within my chest—a longing for that connection. *Show me how*, I prayed.

Soon after that, the Divine Feminine actually started showing up in my house.

I'm not even sure how it happened, but over several months my women friends began to reappear in my life, and my home became a gathering place. Marge was now commuting from Wisconsin to work with me, and stayed with me several nights a week. Karen, my Nurse Practitioner and partner also commuted from Wisconsin to work with me. Roberta—nurse, healer, administrative guru, and friend—commuted from Michigan to work with me one week out of the month. My longtime friend Jeannie (the pastor) worked in Barrington, but had relocated to Wisconsin. Since she worked in Barrington, she stayed with me often. My house began to fill regularly with the warm and loving spirit of women.

I delighted to wake up early, brew my organic, half decaf (water-process) coffee, and carry it to each friend's bedroom door. There was a magic about my home and the conversation and support that happened in the evenings and mornings when these women stayed with me.

My friends started to refer to my house as "Marilyn's B & B."

"Bookings" at the B & B always included Wednesdays, so we usually had at least four or five for dinner those evenings. We cooked together and shared our days and lives. As time went on, other friends began to join us until we had "Women's Wednesdays" at my house every week. It was as if I didn't really live alone.

One Thursday morning, I awoke spontaneously at 5:30, climbed out of bed and headed down the hall to the stairs. Walking past the closed bedroom doors, a warm, cozy feeling surrounded me. My quiet house was alive with women sleeping. As I walked down the stairs, then moved toward the kitchen, I glanced through the doorway to the dining room. A pleasant sensation stirred me. Empty now, the dining room seemed to still hold the congenial vibrations of women around the table, sharing and communing from the night before. Walking over to the island stovetop counter, I started the coffee grinder and put the tea kettle on to heat water. My morning ritual. As I poured the boiling water over the freshly ground coffee beans, a pleasant coffee aroma filled the air. After I poured my mug of coffee, and took the first sip, a sense of satisfaction came over me and I began to replay the previous evening in my mind.

That night there had been four of our five "woo-woo" women present. Our original group was formed when the five of us met at the Barrington Montessori School as young mothers of preschool children twenty-one years earlier. We were drawn together to share something deeper. We were different from one another, but we came together for support and to explore the meaning of life. We learned Tai Chi, explored healing modalities, studied women and their spirituality throughout the ages. We were named the Woo-woos by Jane's sister who was amused by our intense desire to reach out into the cosmos for meaning. We grew up together and were there for all the joys and issues that we faced as mothers, daughters, spouses, and women wanting to make a difference in the world. While our children were young, we met at least once a week, but it had become less frequent over the years.

Until now. Something happens when women gather—especially in midlife. There is a chemistry that cannot be explained, a connection to one another that connects us deeply to ourselves and to the Divine Flow.

As life had gone on, I had lost this lifeline. Work was busy and mothering was time-consuming. My connection to Carl was loosening. Looking back, I had become too tired and perhaps demoralized to keep my connection with my friends, except on occasion. Perhaps I wasn't telling myself the truth, so it was difficult to be with these women who knew me so well—I wouldn't be able to keep myself in the dark...

As we sat together in my dining room the night before, Laura said, "During your marriage, you were like Rapunzel, kept in a tower. Every now and then, you would let down your hair and we could be with you."

Chuckles around the table.

"It is so good to have you back and see you blossoming in your new home and new life," Laura continued. She had been the friend who had tracked with me most closely during those darker years. She would call me, pursue me, persist with me even when I would "go underground" and not connect. She was with me through my ups and downs and trusted me to come through to a better connection with myself.

Now, as I sipped my coffee and breathed in the warm energy from the evening before, peace enveloped me. Belonging. Seen and heard. Connected. I am not alone. As I felt this energy from the night before, I realized we women had created a vessel for the Divine Feminine to flow into our lives and into the world.

I was connecting to a lifeline that had been vital to me as a young mother.

Reconnecting me.

Recovering some lost parts of my soul.

Feeling the glow, I felt myself again in the circle of women. Marge had reminded me of something I'd long forgotten. Some twenty years ago, I had hosted The WiseWoman retreat weekends for mid-life women, empowering them to become their authentic selves as they transitioned into the menopause years. Although I was much younger when I created the program, I had observed the power and depth of wisdom that so many of my patients were able to access at this life stage. For women at midlife, the transition happens on every level: physical, mental, emotional, spiritual, and relational. The WiseWoman retreats were a safe place to explore on all these levels.

As I reflected on those times, a shiver of recognition ran through me. I'd known so much at such a young age but hadn't quite applied it to myself. As I observed women and helped them to reach their full potential in midlife, I was learning from them and preparing myself for my own transition. It seems that I have often had great insight into growth and healing—for others. Exploring women's wisdom and watching women transform had been truly gratifying. Now it was time for me to cultivate my own innate wisdom. Once again: no longer the doctor or the teacher, but the patient, the student.

It made me smile to think of all the women who had touched my life.

Again, as I sat that morning while the other women slept, I recognized once more that the process of healing is an exchange: both the patient and healer gain from the experience. It's an ongoing process that takes time and patience.

My teacher Barbara Brennan once said, "The process of incarnation takes a lifetime."

The Divine Feminine was present in my life.

I was on the way to fully becoming myself.

21. Father of the Bride

I WAS ABOUT TO come full circle, returning home to reconnect in a new way with wisdom I had known long ago.

As the months passed, I felt myself relaxing into a new level of ease. Having the connection to my Wise Women friends supported me to be truly honest and gentle with myself in a way that felt new to me. It was a time filled with insights and fun. I was able to bask in this safety zone, getting healthier and happier for most of a year. It felt as though more of my soul was inhabiting my being. The divine feminine connection was growing within me.

It turns out I had more to discover about my soul's alignment with the masculine.

It was summer when I travelled to Indianapolis to attend my 40th high school reunion. I had connected with a few old friends through email and was looking forward to meeting them again in person. As I drove to the party, I smiled to myself. High school had been a happy time for me, and it dawned on me that I was once again happy. In spite of the difficulties I had been through, I was feeling peaceful, delighted, and radiant. Ready to meet my past.

I had no idea what was in store for me.

Arriving at the welcome table, I was issued a nametag with a photo of my senior picture from high school. Brilliant! These proved enormously helpful it turned out, since many people's looks had really changed. The 1972 North Central High School graduating class had 1,247 people, so I only knew a fraction of them. Though it seemed that I knew almost everyone at this party. Or they knew me. It was heartwarming to connect with friends who had been classmates, and those who worked with me at the Cape Codder Restaurant when I was 17.

"Marilyn, it's you!"

"You haven't changed!

"You look the same."

My younger high school self began to make herself known to me as the evening unfolded. Connecting with these old friends was providing a mirror for me and eliciting my deeper self to come forth. I was recovering that same bright, hopeful young woman that I had been then. The evening was jovial and warm, and somehow, I moved in and out of different groups, discovering more and more connections.

While talking to a couple of women, my friend Todd came from behind and said, "Hey Marilyn, look who I found!"

I turned and my heart leapt. There stood Todd and Rob, our friend. A familiar powerful feeling came over me before my mind registered who it was. Peace started flowing through me. *I have waded into the River again.* Although 35 years had passed since we had last seen one another, it was as if we had never been apart.

When I had dated Rob in high school, it was always powerful. Then and now, in his presence, time was suspended. It was as if we had together entered into a river of peace. Warmth. Gentleness. Eternity. It didn't matter what we were doing, I was in a state of quiet mind and pure Presence. Timeless.

We smiled and hugged simply, then moved easily to a table in the corner where we caught up on each other's lives. We shared stories of our children, his marriage, my divorce, our work. We reviewed the last times we had seen each other—at my college, then at his army base in Texas, and in Chicago.

All the while, we kept bathing in the River, but we never mentioned it...

Finally, when the night was over, as I drove away from the reunion, it occurred to me, *This is Love. Divine Love. My soul is connected to the flow of the Divine.*

Moments from the past played in my mind--moments of being held in Love: with my father, Rob, and other loves in my life. Being with these people somehow made an opening for me to feel fully alive with love.

I began to crave this connection. *I need a partner. Someone who can love me...*

Rob and I began to communicate through email. We talked about the River. He said he wanted to get together again.

Thrilled. Scared.

He was married.

"What are you doing, Rob?" I asked.

"I don't know. I tell my wife everything, but I have not told her about this."

After a long, delicious pause, my rational self spoke, "Be careful please."

We did meet and had a perfect day. Walking and talking and sharing every detail of our lives and hearts. We even took a motorcycle ride like old times. When it was time to say goodbye, we had no regrets. We had maintained a boundary, and I respected Rob for that...

Rob called me an hour after he drove away.

"The most amazing thing happened as I was driving away from you," he said. "A hawk flew down in front of my windshield and looked right at me. Then I glanced over to the side of the road and saw a doe walking out from the trees. As I was driving it occurred to me that the hawk was leaving the doe."

Rob had always been in tune with the natural world. He knew that in Native American wisdom, the deer, especially the doe, is the animal that will lead you to all good things like water, berries and other food, and adventure. The hawk flies high and looks keenly at what is below, able to have a higher perspective.

"I need to be the hawk and as I leave the doe, take a higher perspective," he told me. "There is no doubt you are my Doe, leading me on an adventure to good things."

Smiling to myself, my heart was warmed and all felt right with the world.

But then, as I went through my days, a longing began to grow. Rob and I continued to communicate, and while our conversations were inspiring, afterward there was more of an emptiness in my chest.

Then, as summer wore on, I was not feeling well.

At work one morning, before the patient schedule began, I asked my staff member Janet if she could do a little "emergency healing" on me. As we closed the door to the healing room, a sob grew up in my chest and came out of me. Janet held the energy space open and helped me feel safe to open to a flood of emotions.

"You have been blocking your emotions," she said gently.

I once again realized that I must honor my emotions if I am to open to a true healing. Getting sick was an opportunity to honor my emotions and reach a deeper level of truth with myself.

Later that day, sitting in my meditation chair, I closed my eyes and breathed deeply. Words began to flow into an experience:

Every little ache is a place of holding,
Holding out, holding on.
Every sadness, every pain is a place of tension, remembering a limit,
Grabbing a limitation, hunkering down...

I ask, instead, for my Body, my Beloved Self, to let go
Release the hold and, by letting go,

come upon
Life/Flow/Love.

I awaken into a dream/vision:
    In a beautiful field of grass
    I am walking, hair flowing, long dress flowing. Breeze rustling.
    Smiling, walking, carrying something in my two hands as I walk.
    And from the woods, a man steps out in riding clothes.
    I am carrying something in my hands and reach out to
        return it to him.
It's a bridle.
I nod to him and turn away.
My arms rise up and unfold into wings, I step forward and
then lifting, lifting up, up off ground
    —soaring and flying.
I am. Freedom. Peace. The Dove.

The meditation was a mystery but somehow, I was letting go
of fear and letting go of holding on.
    I gave the bridle back to a man, but I knew I had also imposed
it on myself. The bridle was my own holding back, I must experience my own feelings. I must keep my mind and heart free.

My father, Rob, Carl---the love they have called forth from
me was my connection to Source.
    But I didn't need an intermediary—this River always flows
and I could bathe in it and drink of it without being connected
to a man.
    I choose to open the flow, always.
    Stay connected.
    The partner will appear...

I knew I must completely open my heart to allow the Flow of Love to enliven me, directly. Love with a man can draw me in, dip into the flow, but it is not a substitute for the steady flow of direct Divine Love. Human love is finite. Source Love is infinite.

Summer gave way to fall, and I found myself longing for my Mind and Heart to "make peace in the land" again. About that time, my brother called to tell me of a woman who was doing research using EEG to track states of consciousness and training her subjects to access more meditative and healing brain wave states. Joel, in his usual winning way, had connected with Judith Pennington (the researcher) from his home across the ocean in France to her home/lab in Pennsylvania, and he was in the midst of planning a trip to train with her at a workshop in her home.

"Would you like to join me?" he asked.

Of course, I would!

At that time, Hurricane Sandy was making her way up the east coast. Although I was flying inland of where the hurricane might hit, there were news reports of air travel being crippled and flights cancelled. I spoke to my brother the day before I was to travel and made a decision to leave as soon as possible. He had been working with Judith for five days and insisted that I would not want to miss this opportunity. I called the airline, scrambled to finish packing and made it on a flight one day early. As I bustled into a cab, and rushed off to the airport, I laughed to myself. Only for my brother would I go rushing into a hurricane!

As it turned out, my brother and I were the only two participants who made it to the workshop. A synchrony. We had no idea the depth of experience that awaited us.

It was almost dark when I set out from the airport in a rental car and drove to Judith's home. On the two-hour drive, GPS and my headlights guided me through remote areas of Pennsylvania in the dark. My senses were heightened, and I knew I had started on a journey into the unknown. Finally, as I turned down Judith's lane, I was aware of the huge trees on either side. I drove slowly, because I didn't want to miss the driveway, but also because I felt reverent on this street with its cathedral of trees. I had phoned ahead, so when I arrived, Joel was standing in the driveway to meet me.

"You made it!" he said as he swung open the car door and pulled me into a bear hug.

"We are crazy, aren't we?" I teased.

He helped me gather my things, and we made our way through the garage and into the house.

As I stepped into the large open kitchen, a sense of warmth and peace came over me. My eyes connected with Judith who was standing just inside the door, and we connected with an instant familiarity even before we were introduced, as if we had known each other for ages. We smiled and hugged. Judith's husband, Steve, stepped forward and we greeted each other.

We moved into the warm kitchen and I felt immediately relaxed. Judith started making tea and Joel took me down the central staircase to the lower level where my room was. Joel's room was next door to mine, and our two rooms opened onto a cozy family room. I saw one wall had French doors and picture windows that lined the back wall. On the opposite side of the family room from our bedrooms was another room.

"Come here," Joel lowered his voice and beckoned me as he started to tiptoe toward the room. He paused, eyes dancing, and I had to laugh at his silliness. But of course, this is how we always were. He slowly opened the door to reveal the lab where we would be doing our workshop. There was a desktop in the center of the room with EEG equipment sitting on it, a chair facing the control panel on one side of the desk, and two chairs on the other side for the subjects. I surveyed the set up, and an unexpected feeling of peace and anticipation came over me.

"I can't wait for you to have this experience. It has been incredible," Joel whispered.

When we climbed the stairs back up to the main floor, we noticed a candlelit meal laid out on the tall island counter.

"Judith, how lovely!" I said.

The four of us pulled up tall stools and enjoyed flavorful soup and homemade bread as we got to know one other. Steve is a professor of mathematics and in his quiet way brought an interesting perspective to the brain wave work Judith was doing. Judith first practiced the Mind Mirror technique of brainwave meditation originated by British psychobiologist and biophysicist C. Maxwell Cade in the early 1970s, and later developed into the Awakened Mind program by Anna Wise, Judith's mentor. Anna's health had later deteriorated due to MS, resulting in her death in 2010. Judith further developed the work of the Awakened Mind approach and wrote several best-selling books that taught many to awaken and evolve their minds using EEG Biofeedback Meditation. Judith was approachable and calm, and it slowly dawned on me what an accomplished and influential person she was. She was now a world authority on EEG Meditation who founded an international consortium of awakened mind practitioners.

Joel had told Judith of my work bringing energy healing to medically ill patients, and she wanted to know more. I described to her that as a healer, I would quiet my thoughts and enter a meditative state to be able to sense the energy body that surrounds and supports the physical body. I told her that in that meditative state it was possible to expand consciousness into my own energy body and then discern any blockages or stagnant areas in the chakras or energy fields of my patient. Once the area of concern had been detected, vibrational energy could be directed into the energy body of the patient. This in turn healed the cells of the physical body.

Judith lit up. "I would love to track your EEG state when you expand and do healing!"

"Sounds exciting," I said. I smiled at Joel. He has such a remarkable ability to connect people. I think he even surprises himself.

As we were finishing our dinner, Judith said, "Would you like to do a session tonight?"

I was hoping she would offer!

Steve offered to clean up so the three of us could head down to the lab.

Entering the cozy room, I again felt the calm around me. I settled into one of the comfortable chairs, and Judith and Joel attached EEG leads to my scalp. I would be doing the first exercise and Joel would be assisting Judith. When I was fully wired up, they took their seats at the monitor, and we began.

I closed my eyes and relaxed, ready for an adventure. Listening to Judith's voice, I was led through a series of meditation exercises: recalling a stressful event, feeling empathy, doing mental math, listening to music, visualizing colors. Sometimes I was directed to close my eyes and at other times keep them open. As I followed their voices, they led me from linear thoughts (beta brain waves) into a more peaceful meditative state (alpha) and then back again. Overall, a sense of aliveness and pleasure began to well up in me.

When we finished, they shared the pattern of my brain waves with me, and the drawings and notations were delightful. Judith explained that this first exercise, by practicing moving from beta to alpha states, helps to develop a facility for moving into even deeper states of consciousness by choice.

It was getting late, so we unhooked me from the EEG leads, turned off the equipment, and said our goodnights. Moments later, I happily fell into my cozy bed and into a deep sleep.

When my eyes opened the next morning, I caught my breath. The back yard was actually wooded! Since I arrived in the dark, I had no idea where we were. Beautiful trees cascaded down a gentle hill into a clearing in the distance. Climbing out of bed, a chill ran through me. It was cold! Wrapped up in my cozy robe,

I stepped out into the common room where the woods could be seen through the many picture windows. There also were many branches down and other signs of high winds. Ah, effects of the hurricane. Later when I joined my brother in the kitchen, I learned that there was a power outage. High winds from the distant hurricane had knocked trees into the power wires. From the kitchen window, we could see a fallen tree, six feet in diameter, with its enormous roots exposed. We slept through quite the storm!

It turned out that we were cut off from civilization—no internet and limited phone usage. We cooked on the outdoor grill and stayed mostly in the living room by the big fireplace. In order to begin our journey into the deeper levels of mind, we had to move equipment that was battery operated into the living room where it was warm.

On the second day, we followed as Judith's voice quietly led us from Beta into a meditative Alpha level. Relaxing more deeply, my thoughts slowed and I began to feel an opening, as if entering a large space. My body was very still, and visions and thoughts seemed to appear, as if I were a screen and these creative ideas and pictures were being presented on the screen.

That morning, Judith told us that we would be doing an Animal Sensualization exercise. As we followed Judith's voice prompting the meditation, I began looking to see what animal I would be.

A sleek black panther appeared. Very beautiful. Shifting. A leopard? Unclear. Waiting. Watching.

And then there he was. A lion. Unmovable.

My mind rebelled: This can't be right. Shouldn't I be a lioness? Maybe it will shift again.

The lion was steadfast. Strong. Minutes passed, and he stayed.

Finally, a sense of peace came over me. I accepted the lion.

At first, I watched the lion, and then I became him, and saw from his perspective, as well as observing from a higher perspective. Looking out over a cliff, there was an incredible vast view. Africa. I knew I was the head lion, happy being such a leader of the pride. I had a mate and babies—and cared about the little ones. At one point, there was a moment of vigilance—afraid—knowing that one of my pride had once been shot by a man. Toward the end of the meditation, I saw a glowing light with an orange center. (Judith noted that there was a gamma burst on my brainwaves signaling enlightenment.) During the meditation, Judith had asked what were the qualities of my essence as a lion. Courage. Leadership. Majesty. Power. These filled me and held my whole body in their strength.

When I opened my eyes, I felt the presence and the essence of the lion's qualities within me. To this day, when I need these qualities, I can close my eyes and feel myself as the lion.

He will always be a part of me.

This, I later learned, was the Theta level. It was a whole new world for me, offering resources I never could have imagined. Theta is the subconscious level, a creative state, where we un-leash a wealth of powerful traits, ideas, skills, and insights. It is also the gateway to the deepest level of consciousness, the Delta state. The Delta state allows connection to our unconscious mind. When in the Delta state, I felt no sense of my body, as if I had travelled so deeply within that I was in in touch with the great void where all of creation arises and connects with everything that exists.

By traveling to these inner planes, it was as if the spirit world or dream world could be accessed and made real in this physical world. Insights were abundant.

I first felt a connection with my father at the Delta level, mid-week. Judith had led us in a meditation that reached down to the Theta level.

Traveling down a hallway in a large mansion, I kept coming upon doors. Each one I opened was a bedroom, and inside would be a man that I had known. When I entered the room, the man would disappear behind another door, or I would be unable to get into the room. After several attempts, I found myself back in the hallway and was moved to walk the other direction to the dining room, where there was a large dining table surrounded by many empty chairs. On the wall at the far end of the room was a large mirror. I gravitated to the mirror, and when I peered in, I saw the reflection of the dining room table, but in the mirror, the table was laden with food, and there were people sitting in the chairs. I recognized each person, and they recognized me—each one had died during my lifetime. I looked at each one around the table: Great Aunt Vera, Grandma Mitchell-Goudie, Aunt Vivien, Grandma Huston, Grandpa Huston, my brother Mark, Aunt Bettie, and finally my father.

My father moved to stand before me in the mirror. As we looked at each other, all visible things slowly went out of focus, and we were deeply connected without form. I could feel the strong presence of my father, an expanding energy of pulsing consciousness. I felt his unconditional love and a sense of peace and caring, an essence that was uniquely his.

I felt that I had entered a vast space and this is where my father now existed. Heaven?

Later Judith reported that I was in Delta when I met with my father.

As it was happening, I sensed that I had passed into another place where my father's spirit now existed and he had come forward to meet me. I was receiving an understanding of a vast unconditional Love force that was ever present. My father's spirit now existed in that place and he had come forward to meet me. This felt like the connection I had with him when he was alive, but somehow more vast, and connected to something greater. Source River. His spirit was showing me.

Later, after this experience, when I opened my eyes, I had a deeper understanding of my spiritual nature. It was clear that I had always had a connection to Source, and it had been through my relationship with my father that I felt it most strongly. Somehow, I was looking to connect again through the men in my life, but that didn't last...And then it dawned on me that I felt I would betray the love for my father if I had a partner. Stunned. This was a surprise to me, and it felt important.

In the following days, the spirit of my father was around me as we explored. Several times when Joel and I would awaken from our meditations, we both would report that our father's spirit had been with us. It felt comforting and magical that we had his presence as a guide to the vast Source. It was validating for us both to experience his presence at the same time. This was more than just our imagination.

On the last day, Judith led us into a meditation that shifted everything for me. In the meditation, I walked down a long path that led deep into the woods. A clearing surrounded by deep forest appeared. As I stepped forward into the clearing, a sense of peace came over me. I waited, and after some time a tall man dressed in pharaoh's garb emerged from the trees opposite and walked toward me, stopping before me. As I looked up into his eyes, a recognition ran through me: This is my partner. My true partner. As we stood there, I realized I was an Egyptian queen. Next, the men from my life, all my lovers from all time, stepped forward from the woods around us, to honor us and witness this union, and formed a circle around us.

As we stood in this peaceful circle, I sensed the spirit of my father above and around us. I heard these words from my father: "You honor me by this union with your true partner. And now, in this way you allow me to finally become Father of the Bride." With this, I felt a warm wave descend over us, like a blanket of peace. A blessing. And then wave after wave. Blessing upon blessing.

As I emerged from this mediation, I knew I had forged a new relationship with my father, and with myself. I had made space to have my right partner, and I connected directly with the vast River of Unconditional Love.

On that fifth day, after the meditation, the power came back on at Judith and Steve's home. It seemed appropriate as we left our retreat and headed back into the bustling world.

As we drove off to the airport, Joel and I marveled at what had transpired. We had shared a journey that opened our soul connection in a new, deeper way.

How to flow life force and mindfulness through my body and
   my life?
Love with a man?
   Love opens to the River
   Unconditional

Overwhelming peace and light
   Flowing in my feet, my womb, my breasts, my heart, my hands
   Soaking up, pooling—
   Throat, brain, sinuses
   Flowing along the river of my spine
Breath eases the direction of the flow
   Gentle direction
   More love in waves
Breath holds the note for physical structure
   Guides the flow into a form...
   Juicy form, pulsing

Marrying and mediating the cage of hard thoughts
Softening and expanding so thought has life force—
Cage becomes a flexible container

Where am I?
Slowing movement
Ease of deep breaths
Deeply within the body
Deeper, deeper
To touch the vast inner/outer space...
All is here—the multipotent void.
I AM.
So be it.

I now felt I had accessed the Divine feminine, and aligned my relationship to men, and somehow, I was reorganizing, becoming more whole.

22. Finding my Voice

I WAS DIFFERENT.

Somehow, more present, more centered. *Grounded.* Yet lighter. *Connected and expanded.*

I knew that I had made a profound shift in my way of being, and I wanted to understand. At my first opportunity, I met myself in my meditation chair, closed my eyes, and relaxed. *What do I need to know?*

The predictable calm washed over me and I waited.

I was taken back to the time before my cancer diagnosis, and I began to review my healing journey. Looking at myself then, a great compassion arose in me for the busy, harried doctor I once was. I had known for a long time that energy healing offered the promise to patients of a more complete recovery and greater wellbeing than expected—even better health than before the illness—and I wanted that for my patients. Now, as a doctor, a healer, and a patient myself, I saw how energy healing supported medical treatments, especially in cases where there was little or nothing to offer, or when medical treatments were not working. My team of healers and I witnessed astounding results in our healing patients. We were making a difference. Breaking new ground.

Healing was moving but it was also exhausting. Then, everything changed. It wasn't until energy healing failed to eradicate my cancer that I started on a journey to learn the true nature of healing. Looking back, I realized that until that moment, I had been using healing as a *technique*, like surgery or medicines, or physical therapy.

Healing is not a technique. Healing is *a connection.*

That message was now loud and clear. Before my cancer diagnosis, I'd used healing energy in my work with patients, and my patients successfully made their own connections to spirit, all without my own consciousness shifting. Funny how we healers can facilitate profound healing in others, and even witness their strong connections to heart, soul, and life force, but not necessarily make those connections for ourselves.

So, when healing *as a technique* failed, it got my attention.

I learned to let go and listen, and my connection grew stronger. Looking back over my own journey, it was obvious that each step had been divinely orchestrated to bring me to this understanding. When I would relax, open, and trust, the next step in my healing process would appear. Keeping my heart open was key.

I was now forging a more consistent connection to spirit. Previously, I was trying to use or control the energy, but that only went so far. When I let go of control and connected to something greater, the energy was *unharnessed.* I could now work in a more expansive dimension —beyond just the mind. A sense of awe ran through me. *This connection to Spirit/Energy has always been with me. When I connect rather than control, I have an unlimited Source to draw upon.*

I felt an overwhelming sense of gratitude, and then heard these words:

Create a life
Create a book
  Bring forth inspiration

Live with Radiance
Open the Flow
One's life story is full of
   Source light
      Reaching down
         Lightening!
           Lighting up
              Flooding the body
And still
   It can be drained away
   Become small, rigid,
Back in the cage
though the door is wide open
Must remember
   To breathe
    Relax
Letting go dissolves the cage
Breathing brings the flow

With the obstacles removed
  Unconditional love walks in...
   Pure Love

I step into my new role
New Life

Coming into my own

Life, Work, Love

in full Radiance,
   Brilliance
      Service

⟋

I opened my eyes and was practically bursting with excitement.

The source of true healing, the Life Force, is pure, unconditional love. I had learned that one must be completely open to their own heart's truth in order to allow the flow of Love Energy to fully enliven the body.

As I contemplated this, I had an overwhelming desire to share my knowledge with everyone, including my fellow doctors. *I need to take my approach out from behind closed doors and onto a larger platform. This could change medical care.*

How could I get Healing and Medicine, which have been separate for so long, to come together? I decided to trust that the next steps and opportunities would present themselves, but I never could have predicted the path.

Just as I was making this shift, my medical practice at WomanCare began to shift. From the beginning of my medical practice, the holistic, natural, and alternative practices I studied were incorporated with the medical care I was trained to give. Five years earlier I had taken the exam to become board certified in Integrative Medicine, which identifies and certifies doctors who have competence in blending medicine and holistic measures in their practice.

At the office, I began to be inundated with patients seeking energy healing and medical care. New patients were seeking help with problems that were not readily solved by medical care alone or diagnoses that had failed medical treatments. My returning patients were embracing energy healing and referring their family members and friends.

The demand was growing. Doctors began to take notice and sent us referrals. I continued making referrals to the same medical colleagues as I always had, and now these doctors were beginning to ask me about the healing; they observed improvements in the recovery of their patients that received our healing treatments, and my patients were telling their doctors about our approach.

One fearful, anxious patient was offered hip replacement surgery due to severe degeneration that caused difficulty walking and extreme pain. Her first hurdle was actually scheduling the procedure. After some urging, she began to work with a Healing Practitioner and agreed to the operation. The patient was comforted knowing that she would have distance energy healing during her surgical procedure. Afterward, she surprised herself and her doctor by recovering much more quickly than expected. When her doctor expressed surprise at her astounding recovery, she told him about her energy healing sessions. This patient was so happy with her outcome, when her sister was diagnosed with the same condition, she referred her to the same surgeon and the same Healing Practitioner. Again, the doctor was astounded when the sister had a similar recovery, and he mentioned it to me.

I had his attention, and was getting used to having other doctors' attention, too, though they were surprised and puzzled. They all wanted to understand more about what was going on.

❧

One Sunday afternoon, one of our patients gave us a surprising opportunity.

I was in my kitchen at home when the phone rang. It was Tricia, and she told me our patient May was scheduled for surgery the next day with Dr. Loren. May wanted Tricia to be in the operating room to do healing, and Tricia was hoping I could help make this possible.

May first came to me a year earlier with an abdominal hernia reporting that she had undergone two repair surgeries, both of which had failed. She wanted to try energy healing. I referred her to Tricia for healing sessions and May experienced temporary closure of the hernia. But after a week, the closure didn't hold. This happened several times. Surgery was the next step.

.

Tricia had performed numerous healings during surgery, but always at a distant location. This would be her first time in the actual operating suite.

I called Dr. Loren's answering service, knowing it was probably a long shot. Even though Dr. Loren was not on call, he called me right back. I presented the idea of having my healer in the OR and promised to escort her and be there for the surgery.

"Sure, Marilyn. Whatever you want."

"You are the best, Al."

I hung up the phone and called the OR desk next. I explained the situation and that Dr. Loren was in favor of having my healer in the OR. After numerous phone calls back and forth, we got approval!

The following morning, Tricia met me in the women's surgery locker room. She informed me that another patient of hers was in the hospital and was scheduled for surgery later in the morning. She was hoping to be in on that case, too. Yikes. I didn't know the surgeon—we had already stretched the rules with this.

We exchanged our clothes for surgical scrubs and made our way out to the surgical hallway. At the central surgery desk, we checked in with the Surgical Coordinator, and were informed that our patient would soon be in Room 14. I mentioned to the Coordinator that there was another patient scheduled for surgery today who wanted Tricia in the OR with her. The Coordinator agreed to check with the surgeon.

Walking down the hall to OR 14, Tricia and I talked over the plan. When we arrived, the staff was preparing the OR.

"Hi Dr. Mitchell!"

"Hi, everyone! This is Tricia Eldridge, master healer. She will be doing energy healing while Dr. Loren operates."

It was clear that the staff had been forewarned and there was excitement in the air. I found a place for Tricia to work that was away from the surgical field, and out of the surgeon's line of sight. I didn't want him to be distracted.

Slowly, the room filled in. All the packs were open, and the patient was wheeled in and helped onto the OR table. Soon the anesthesiologist appeared to begin his work. Finally, the surgeon arrived.

In the operating room, the surgeon calls all the shots. When Dr. Loren walked through the door, the air in the room shifted. *Respect for Dr. Loren. He is open to this unique opportunity and we are all proud of him.* After checking in with the room and the staff, he slipped out the door to scrub at the sink. *Quiet. Expectant.*

Dr. Loren came back through the door and approached the scrub nurse at her table. A sterile towel was transferred to the doctor and he dried his hands. Snap! The paper gown unfolded to full length and the nurse held it for the doctor while he pushed his arms through. Snap! One glove on, then the other. The circulator tied the back of his gown, and he tied the front. Ready to go!

Dr. Loren moved around the OR table to get into position to operate. Tricia and I adjusted our position so the healing wouldn't distract him. As he passed us, he said, "So, is there any science behind this energy healing?" There was playfulness in his voice.

"Yes, there is, Doctor!" I shot back at him. "We will talk."

Dr. Loren moved close in beside the patient and focused his attention into the narrow world of his surgical field. *Concentrating.*

As he worked, Tricia began her work, moving her fingers in tiny, rapid movements. Quiet, laser focus energy.

As the procedure progressed, the air lightened. Dr. Loren spoke to his team. Occasionally, Tricia spoke to me. Staying by her side, I let Tricia know what the surgeon was doing. From my perspective, watching both work, a subtle dance between them became apparent. Tricia restructured organs after Dr. Loren cut them. Tricia "suctioned" energetically, then Dr. Loren suctioned physically. There was an intricate interplay between surgeon and healer, both doing the same surgery but on two different planes.

The entire team felt part of this moment. The air was jovial. *It's intriguing to them.* We felt part of something greater.

So often during surgery, we narrow our awareness to the task at hand. Focus and attention are important. The sterile and safety routines are important. We get good at our respective jobs and come together to do a procedure that will benefit the patient. More slick and efficient than repairing a car. We take pride in creating a good result.

It is the rare moment, the rare surgery, when we remember that we are also between the worlds: holding someone in the state between life and death and performing a sacred dance on their behalf. Whether aware or not, this is the place we enter when we participate in surgery.

For this surgery, I was in the unique position of witness to a meeting of both worlds.

Finally, the surgery was winding down. Dr. Loren and Tricia finished at the same time. The spell was broken: drapes were pulled off of the patient and discarded, the surgeon moved away to pull off his gown and gloves, the patient moved as she awoke from anesthesia. The hush was broken. Nurses started discussing who was going on break.

Dr. Loren walked over to us.

"Everything went well," he said.

"Thank you so much for having me in the room," Tricia said.

"Any time."

As we prepared to leave the OR, the head nurse stepped in to inform us that the surgeon on the next case probably did not want a healer in the OR. Ugh. Darn. Since I didn't know the surgeon, it was understandable.

"Well, Trish. I will see you at the office when you finish. If you can't be in on the surgery, you can work with the patient from a distance at the office."

Later I learned that Dr. Loren spoke to the surgeon who was refusing to have a healer in the OR. After telling him it was "no big deal, not a problem," the surgeon changed his mind and he allowed Tricia into the OR. A pancreatic Whipple procedure typically takes him seven hours to complete. With a healer present, it took him 3.5 hours!

After that, he told Tricia he would have her in his OR any time.

We began to have more and more patients requesting healings. Our need for healers was increasing. I decided to establish HealingSpace, an initiative to bring healers into the office to work.

Three of the healers travelled in from Michigan to do healings in the office. Tricia, our teacher, Roberta, and Susie drove in for a week every month and were scheduled in our office with healing appointments for that week. Audrey was our healer who lived locally and came in two days every week to work.

Only Roberta was medically trained, and it became apparent that there needed to be more training for our other healers. Their healing skills were excellent, but their comfort level translating the healing into something understandable to patients and medical personnel was another matter. Roberta had a background in nursing and medical administration. She and I started offering a weekend workshop to transition healers into the medical setting.

We had six more healers who wanted to come to work in our medical office. Although I was thrilled at the prospect of bringing more healers on staff, this presented some problems. WomanCare's facility couldn't accommodate that many healers, and it was becoming clear that they also needed on-going training. With the potential of ten healers, this seemed like an enormous project.

At the same time, I had been considering curtailing my gynecology practice to offer more time to my Integrated Medicine practice for patients seeking solutions that weren't being satisfied by traditional medicine alone.

After much deliberation, I knew what I had to do. After 27 years as a practicing gynecologist, it was time to move on to my new calling and my own practice. HealingSpace moved into its own location and became an Integrated Medical & Healing practice as well as a resource and educational initiative. I approached Marge to see if she would join me working at Healing-Space, and I was elated when she agreed.

Roberta and I decided to create a year-long internship for our healers to provide the on-going training and support that they needed. During this internship, the healers would become Healing Practitioners, able to participate on a medical team with other medical professionals in a variety of medical settings.

My dream was starting to become a reality! Medicine and healing were now integrated in our practice and changing the landscape of choices for patients.

Launching HealingSpace was a big first step in bringing healing and medicine together. We started seeing patients with complex illnesses, offering them integrated medicine approaches and energy healing. By addressing the many dimensions of health, and designing natural and medical treatment plans while guiding patients to shift from their limiting patterns of thoughts and behaviors to their own intuitive powers, we began to have profound results. The response to this dual approach was tremendous. We had the privilege of witnessing many patients transform after struggling for years. Word spread and our practice grew.

We began a Healer's Internship, meeting once a month for a daylong conference and supervising Healing Practitioners between sessions, but it still felt like we were just scratching the surface of what was possible. I was itching to have a wider influence and to bring my message to more patients and physicians than just my small circle. I felt we were on the verge of something greater.

It was again a patient who catalyzed our next leap.

Three years earlier my patient Judy began her journey with cancer. I remember when I saw her name on my patient list. She had been my patient for over a decade—wiry and hyper, and such a sweetheart. But she always seemed pressured. I always did my best to infuse calm into the room. She had been diagnosed with ovarian cancer, and I remember thinking, *She will surely be off the wall today.* This wonderful woman, a nurse by training, had studied natural and alternative methods to support health, and it bothered her that she couldn't quiet her anxiety. She tried relaxation techniques, yoga, meditation, all of which had worked temporarily, but then her racing thoughts would return. It was a vicious cycle of anxiety about her anxiety.

When I entered the examination room, expecting she'd be a wreck, I saw Judy sitting in the chair and I paused. *The room was strangely calm.* Our eyes met. *She was peaceful.*

"Dr. Mitchell, I have ovarian cancer," she stated simply.

I already knew as I'd seen the report.

"I'm so sorry," I said.

"You know, it's odd, but I just think it's going to be OK. Somehow, all the anxiety that I was having, always worrying that something bad was going to happen to me. Now that something has happened, I feel calmer. I have ovarian cancer and I feel calm and clear and I intend to be fine. Isn't that strange?"

I looked into her eyes. "It's remarkable," I said. "Your attitude will truly help you, and I will stand by you through this process."

After reviewing her reports and examining her, we discussed her next steps. Judy had heard of Dr. Julian Schink, the Chief of Gynecological Oncology at Northwestern Medicine, and I heartily supported her choice of specialist. I contacted him to present her case details. Funny, I knew him from when he was just a resident and fellow in training (in those days we called him "Skip"), and now he was the Medical Director of the Cancer Center at Northwestern. She would get excellent medical care.

Then, I wondered if Judy would be open to energy healing? It could really help.

"Judy, would you be interested in working with an Energy Healing Practitioner? I have a very accomplished healer here today who has worked with cancer. I could introduce you."

Judy's response was overwhelming. "Oh, Dr. Mitchell. Yes! I'd be open to that."

"You are going to do very well," I said.

"Dr. Mitchell, I hope to have a miracle."

Audrey, the healer, was standing in the hall when Judy and I walked out of the exam room together. I introduced them, then walked Judy up to the front desk to schedule a healing with her.

After Judy left, I told Audrey of Judy's advanced ovarian cancer.

Audrey looked alarmed.

"That's so serious," she said. "I have never worked on such a serious cancer."

I reassured her that the gyne oncologist and I would also be seeing Judy.

"I know you will be great," I said. "I believe in you."

Judy approached her healing with enthusiasm. She decided to undergo a detox and started a clean and healthy diet. She educated herself about supplements, and we put together a regimen that was immune boosting and nourishing. She was doing everything to support herself.

She saw Dr. Schink, who ordered the scans and testing to find out if the cancer had spread. While this workup was going on, she scheduled regular visits with me to support her on her therapies, and began a series of energy healing sessions.

Her anxiety returned intermittently, and during our regular visits we worked with techniques to reclaim that deep calm that she had once experienced. One of her visits with me really stood out. We reviewed her diet and supplement regimen, which seemed to be working well for her. Then we reviewed her workup: scans revealed that the cancer was widespread in her abdominal cavity, including tumors that wrapped around the bowel and a nodule in her lung. This indeed confirmed Stage IV cancer, and Judy was told that her initial surgery would include removal of the involved bowel, as well as hysterectomy, omentum removal, lymph node dissection, and general tumor debulking. Because of the severity and widespread involvement, she was being scheduled for pre-op chemo in order to reduce tumor size prior to surgery.

Despite this news, Judy was surprisingly calm. And then she said, "I have been having some amazing healings with Audrey, and I believe they will help me have a good outcome."

This patient was feeling more confident about the process than I was!

"In the last healing, I saw an angel, Judy said. "He turned his back on me and waved me away, kicking up dust as he left. He said quite clearly, I don't want you. Audrey told me it must have been the Angel of Transition."

I knew the Angel of Transition was an emanation healers sometimes see if the person was close to death.

I was stunned—and instantly felt better. But ovarian cancer is tricky. I was glad my doubts weren't contagious. She was better off keeping all her peaceful positive thoughts in place.

Finally, the day arrived for Judy's surgery. She had been given pre-op chemotherapy and the results of her CA125 tumor test were much better. Her doctor was pleased by this marked response and surprised that she tolerated the chemo so well. (Judy hadn't told him that she was doing healing.) Judy was informed that, during the surgery, she would have all visible tumor removed, including the involved part of her bowel, and would possibly require a colostomy.

On the day of the surgery, Audrey was in the office doing a long-distance healing on Judy, tracking the surgery, and helping things to go smoothly. Late in the morning, Audrey came running down the hall and burst into the conference room where I was finishing my morning charting.

"There's no cancer! They opened her and it was gone!" She was beaming.

"No *visible* cancer," I corrected. "Amazing. We will wait for the pathology to see the extent. So, they didn't take out her bowel?"

"No. They couldn't see any to remove. Her husband called me."

We hugged each other. "Oh my gosh, it worked again!" we said together. Although we as healers believe in the energy healing and have seen its amazing effects frequently, it still feels like a miracle when something so profound happens.

It was indeed true, there was no visible cancer in her abdomen: not on the bowel, not on the ovaries, the omentum, or the pelvic sidewalls. The surgeons had been able to perform a simpler surgery than originally planned, removing the uterus, ovaries, omentum, and lymph nodes. A scan revealed that even the lung nodule had disappeared!

But what did they find microscopically? Standing by the FAX machine later that week, I pulled each page off to read as it printed. *Astounding.* Even though it was written in pathology lingo, there was amazement between the lines. "Despite multiple sections...only detached sheets of cancer cells...no cancer... small focus of cancer..." Just the most minimal amount of cancer was found.

After she recovered from surgery, Judy came to my office for a visit.

"You had your miracle, Judy, just like you planned. No visible cancer at your surgery!" I beamed.

"So, it's true then." Tears rimmed her eyes. Judy relayed that after surgery, when she was still recovering from anesthesia, she overheard her family saying something about no more cancer, but she dismissed it. She was shielding herself from disappointment in case it wasn't true. She just didn't dare believe it could happen to her. When I shared the pathology report with her, she was visibly moved. This was the first moment she let the information in.

Later, when Judy saw Dr. Schink for a checkup, he said to her, "I have never seen anything like this. This is an incredible response to pre-op chemo!"

"Well, I had a healer working with me," she finally revealed.

Northwestern had been offering massage-healing sessions to their cancer patients. "You mean one of our healers?" he asked.

"No. One of Dr. Mitchell's healers."

"I will have to talk to Dr. Mitchell!"

Judy had very few side effects with her post op chemo treatments, and she became the poster child for ovarian cancer recovery. She finished therapy and began travelling with her husband and enjoying life.

"I am happier and healthier than I was before," she told me.

One year after she finished her treatments, Judy called to tell me that her CA125 cancer marker was creeping up slowly on a recent blood test. Although no evidence of tumor could be found on her scans, there was a concern that some of the cancer was creeping back in. Her oncologists were observing her and considering some more rounds of chemo.

Judy scheduled a series of healings with Audrey.

After her first healing, Audrey stopped me in the hallway at the office.

"Judy is amazing. When she finished her initial treatments, she went off to enjoy life with her husband. You can't blame her. The only problem is that she let go of her self-care, self-awareness and gratitude, almost like she was defying the cancer rather than respecting it. We learned all this in her recent healing. She has her awareness back."

Judy went through several more rounds of chemo, and a series of healings, reinforcing her commitment to complete well-being. Again, she experienced very few side effects from the chemo. Her CA125 reduced to normal, and she did well.

During a visit with me during that time, she asked if Dr. Schink had contacted me. He hadn't.

"That's surprising," she said, "because he mentions you every time I see him."

That lit me up! At that point, I had four cancer patients seeing Dr. Schink and doing energy healings as well. All were in remission. He must have noticed.

After Judy's visit, I made a beeline for my office and called Dr. Schink's administrator. She put me right through to him.

"Marilyn! I hear about this great work you are doing," he said. "Would you be willing to come and meet with me so we could discuss it?"

Would I? I almost dropped the phone. "That would be great, Skip!"

We arranged a meeting for the following week.

When I arrived at his office, I checked in with his secretary. He immediately appeared at his office doorway and ushered me in. He looked stately and professional in his white lab coat, but his broad grin and dancing eyes betrayed him as the mischievous boy he had been two and a half decades before when we were both young doctors.

Skip toured me through the newest facility of the Northwestern Lurie Comprehensive Cancer Centers devoted to women's cancers. It was a beautiful facility, with rooms and features that were designed for the peace and comfort of women patients. I raved about his facility, and he beamed like a proud papa.

I shared my dream of bringing Energy Healing Practitioners into a medical setting to partner more closely with doctors. I had brought along the data that we were collecting on our patients and the surprising results we were getting. We looked over the results together, and what he saw intrigued him.

"These results are impressive enough to consider a pilot study on cancer patients. We have some studies published on the benefit of alternative therapies for patient symptoms, but nothing about a healing modality like this that may be impacting the course of the disease."

Dr. Schink was enthusiastic about the possibilities and offered to set up a meeting with his Administrator and Research Coordinator to look at the feasibilities of doing a study.

As I left our meeting, a feeling of delight ran through me. *I have reconnected with a friend and now have an ally in academic medicine. All it took was sharing who I am.*

What a confirmation!

I went back to our Healing Practitioners bursting with the news that the Chief of Gyne Oncology and Medical Director of the Cancer Center at Northwestern found our results research-worthy.

And then, as if orchestrated by divine plan, cancer patients began to find us. Friends, relatives, and associates of ours from across the country called to introduce their neighbor, friend, or colleague who had recently been diagnosed with cancer, always with the same message, "I really want them to get the benefit of your energy healing."

Soon each of our Healing Interns had one or two cancer patients, most of them long-distance. At our monthly meetings, the interns reported on their patients using the same language and presentation template that is used in medicine. In this way, we developed a way for medicine and healing to communicate with one another.

Skip and I had several meetings to discuss our possible collaboration. One meeting in particular really opened a new door.

We were sitting in Skip's office when he wheeled around from his computer and looked me in the eyes.

"You know, what you do is Survivorship! Survivorship is the hot new topic for oncology, and it is really in its early stages--the current new frontier in cancer treatment. Because more and more people are living beyond their cancer treatments, it has been recognized that these patients need special attention. For the most part, the care has focused on making sure patients keep up with their cancer screenings and are educated and screened for additional problems they may develop due to the treatments they received. But you have been doing Survivorship all along, in a truly comprehensive way."

I started researching Survivorship programs. National guidelines were being developed. Some programs offered more support to patients in terms of psychological counseling, nutrition, or occupational support. But this varied from institution to institution. What we were doing was more thorough and offered a whole new dimension to recovery and well-being. We were helping people to engage with their life force.

"What you're doing is really the ultimate in Survivorship!" Skip had said.

I was stunned. At first, I couldn't speak. As he said those words, an energy opened around me connecting like a column of light from heaven to earth. I heard the words: *You will be a healer of the system.*

Cancer is the most frightening and difficult of health issues facing medicine right now. Cancer survivorship is a place where we truly could make a difference. And this amazing soul connection of survivorship is not only a path for cancer patients but one for everyone. Everyone can benefit from what we learn with cancer.

Cancer is the Great Teacher
Here now at the door
Ominous,
    Awesome,
        Terrible
And yet—full of Power

Open the door
    Face this conundrum
      Face down the fear
Open the door
Feel the power and light
    That dissolves fear, doubt, holding out
Transmute this cancer
    And be set free.
Connect through heart, past Cancer to the Source.
No separation from the love of God.

23. Connection: The True Nature of Healing

AS OUR WORK EXPANDED, we continued to have more and more success stories of patients getting profound results and feeling that they were more alive in the process. All of our patients had integrative medical treatments in combination with the healing. It felt as if the connection between medicine and healing was truly deepening.

I will never forget the final day of our year-long Healers Intern Training Program. When it came time for Case presentations, I sat in my chair at the front of the group and looked out at the semicircle of healers before me. My eyes met Roberta's, and we smiled. *These healers have become so professional. They are ready to participate in a medical setting.*

Janet presented first. Her patient, Liz, had been diagnosed with Stage IV breast cancer four months earlier. Her doctors did not offer surgery because the tumor was too large, and there were metastases to her bones and liver. She was not offered radiation therapy either. In the end, Liz was treated with chemotherapy. During the months she was undergoing her medical treatment, Liz began doing weekly healings with Janet. Because Liz lived on the East coast, and Janet was in Chicago, all of their healing sessions were conducted at a distance.

"As you recall, the patient had an unexpectedly dramatic response to her chemotherapy, with all of her tumors regressing. She had a procedure to cauterize the now small spot of tumor on her liver, and her bone tumors became undetectable. Her breast tumor had regressed to a size small enough that the doctors offered her a lumpectomy, and low dose radiation therapy, as they would for a Stage I patient. They told Liz that this was the first time they had seen a response like this."

A ripple of excitement ran through the circle. (My medical mind raced: *the doctors did not expect her to do so well, and were inspired by her result.*)

Janet continued: "She had clear margins after her lumpectomy, and negative lymph nodes. Three weeks ago, all of her scans were repeated, and the doctors have declared her cancer free."

We listened, and as our attention was held by Janet's story, our circle of healers was connecting our energy. *It feels like a deep YES.* It is the place where we feel miracle, even as we trust that this healing is always available.

"You know," Janet said, "the most gratifying thing is the way Liz has shifted in her comfort with life, and with her authentic self. When we first started the healing sessions, Liz told me how she had just made a move to a temporary home before she was diagnosed with cancer. She was already stressed and overwhelmed by the move and feeling disconnected and unsupported in her marriage. She loved being a mother to her three daughters but had also been feeling resentment about how much of her time had to be devoted to parenting, which of course made her feel guilty.

"Through our healing sessions, she got in touch with deep unconscious feelings of being unfulfilled. Liz felt a profound sadness for humanity and a sense that she was supposed to make a big contribution to humanity using creative energy. She was plagued by a sense of 'running out of time'.

"We worked on her deep emotions, and as she learned to stay in the moment and reframe her views of her world and relationships, she became peaceful and developed a strong spiritual connection.

"It was remarkable to see how her personal growth and freedom paralleled the cancer regression. She has a more satisfying marriage and even moved into a permanent home that she loves."

The room was reverently silent.

"Janet, that is amazing work," I breathed.

"Liz made a great turnaround on many levels. She now is aware that fears are coming up for her about recurrence, but she has developed enough awareness to stop, reframe and stay in the present. I am so happy for her," Janet said.

Gwen presented next:

"My patient is a 75-year-old woman who was diagnosed with Stage II bladder cancer. She had surgery to remove the tumor, and because the left ureter was compromised, she also had reconstruction with stent placement in that ureter. Intraoperative, the surgeon performed a chemotherapy wash of the bladder. Energy Healing was also performed at a distance during her surgery.

Although the surgery was considered successful, the patient experienced inordinate pain post-operatively. Gwen was instrumental in helping the patient with her unremitting pain.

"We had three healing sessions post-op, but the first one was the most dramatic. At five days post-op the patient still experienced unremitting pain. As we started the healing, I was able to send vibrations that eased the pain while I worked. What was apparent to me was that the pain was emanating from both the ureter and the bladder. The ureter was constantly contracting trying to "move" the surgical injury, as it would to pass a kidney stone. Because there was nothing to move (except perhaps the stent), the pain was unrelenting. The bladder was irritated from the chemotherapy wash."

"As I was working with the surgical site to heal these tissues and cells, a scene opened up that represented trapped energy in the tissues. The patient "saw" herself as a soldier on a cot who had been injured in combat and had some emergency attention, but part of her abdomen was still open. The pain was intolerable. As we held the visual of this, it became softer and a strong, pure light energy began to pour into the wound and then through her entire body. After some time, the whole scene dissolved and there was just pure light.

"After that healing, the patient had no more pain."

Again, we were drawn in.

"That is wonderful, Gwen," I said.

"We continued to work, and after her third healing, the doctors said that she was healed enough to have the stent removed. They had intended to leave it in for three to six months and couldn't explain why her healing had been so rapid."

We smiled.

"This patient is still cancer free."

Laura was next to present. Tami is Marge's neighbor, and Marge had referred her to us for healing when she was diagnosed with Stage III pancreatic cancer. Laura met with Tami over the phone soon after her diagnosis and was able to work with her throughout the entire course of her treatment.

"Tami and I have just finished our sixth energy healing session. When she first came to me, her intention was to decrease her fear and anxiety and be more like her old self. Her history includes a Whipple procedure to remove the cancer, from which she has fully recovered, with all abdominal tubes removed and an increased appetite. During the Whipple procedure, she suffered a stroke, from which she has also recovered. Her physical balance is now normal, her memory has increased, her thinking is clear, and she has had return of vision in the right eye, which had disappeared as a result of the stroke.

"She is now doing beautifully. She walks three to five miles twice a week, she attended her son's wedding and felt like her old self, and she has released much of her fear and anxiety. She wants to learn meditation to keep her heart and mind clear and less fearful. At the end of the sessions she was peaceful, hopeful, and grateful.

"Her doctors have declared her to be in remission and cancer free."

Amazement washed over the group.

After a moment, Marge broke the silence by saying, "Tami has had an amazing response to this healing work. When it was time for her first healing session, she was nauseous to the point that she wanted to reschedule the session. At Laura's encouragement she went ahead with the session and she no longer had nausea symptoms by the end of the hour. This really helped her to engage in the healing connection and get great benefit from these sessions."

"This work is such a blessing!" Laura said.

Next around the circle was Sue. She had been working with Linda who was diagnosed with Stage III pancreatic cancer.

"I am presenting an update on Linda, whom you recall had healings along with her medical treatment. Initially her doctors designed an aggressive and strenuous chemotherapy for her, her particular combination being an experimental protocol. She had extreme fatigue and some other side effects, but much fewer than expected by her doctors, so they continued their course of chemo longer than usual.

"After her chemotherapy treatment was complete, she began a course of intense radiation therapy. We continued her healing sessions and she sailed through the first half of her radiation treatment without side effects. Until one day. She had a checkup with her doctors, and they told her that they were concerned because they had expected her to have some intense side effects with these doses of radiation. After that, she took a down turn and began to have side effects. At her next healing, I pointed out the timing of her side effects and we worked to get her unhooked from buying into the doctors' expectations. After that she completed her RT without an issue. That episode was important for her to feel empowered about her health.

"Anxiety was an issue for her, and we continued to work on that through the entire course of her treatment. She made a profound discovery during our healing sessions. Her mother had some serious psychological problems, and Linda had suffered emotional and physical abuse during her childhood. She did some very effective psychological counseling work and felt at peace with this. As the healing work continued, it became apparent that there still were blockages in her body from emotions suppressed so early and so deeply that they couldn't be reached by the counseling. In fact, her abdomen was essentially 'blocked with cancer'. This made sense to Linda, and after releasing these suppressed emotions, she said she felt 'truly free'. She was able to deeply let go of the past and make a profound shift in connection.

"Linda has been declared cancer free for some time now. She was able to vacation with her husband without undue fatigue, and she is free of anxiety. We are working on the neuropathy that is still present, and it is slowly improving."

As Sue finished her presentation, the room was silent. Another person had made the deep connection, and hearing her story connected us, too.

After some time, Jill spoke. She was working with Joy, a patient who was diagnosed with an aggressive familial form of Endometrial Cancer.

"Joy is a patient who was diagnosed with Stage III endometrial cancer at age 35. Her initial cancer surgery included a complete hysterectomy with lymph node dissection. She also had a long course of chemotherapy, followed by a course of Radiation therapy. She has a history of Lupus and Hypothyroidism. Three years after her cancer diagnosis, she was found to have Myasthenia Gravis, and she had another surgery to remove her thymus gland.

"As if that weren't enough, when she was a teenager, her parents were brutally murdered one evening in a fast food restaurant that they owned. Joy was working that evening but had left work early. She had been fighting with her mother. So, she has had some major emotional trauma.

"When we started our healing sessions, Joy was in the middle of her medical treatment. It was difficult to make a connection with her, but I knew that is what she needed the most—connection. In the first session, there were many cellular memory releases from suppressed emotions. At one point, I even heard the spleen screaming---as if it was venting anger. Joy had survivor's guilt and feelings of unworthiness. She always needed to be in control, so her feelings wouldn't overwhelm her. She seemed to have an inability to let go and allow herself to rejuvenate.

"It was hard for Joy to connect, and she was self–critical. It took time, but in the end, she has truly been able to find herself. She is relaxed and directed and she has shed a lot of her past trauma. She is starting to live up to her name 'Joy'.

"She has been cancer free for five years."

A ripple of delight moved through our circle.

Maureen looked up and chuckled. She was the last healer to present. "Well, here we go..."

"My patient Bonnie is a 78-year-old woman who came to me after she had a recurrence of Malignant Melanoma of the thigh. She had surgery to remove the lesion, but when the pathology came back, the margins were not free of cancer. In addition, she had a suspicious lymph node on one of her scans. She was told by her doctors that there was no more treatment available for her. When I met her she said, 'Maureen, it's you and me.'

"Our first three healing sessions were over the phone, and then we met for a healing in person. She was experiencing edema at that time. All in all, we did seven healings before she went to California for the winter. She had her scans repeated and they came back all clear! Her edema had abated too.

"She has been declared cancer free for over a year now. The doctors were very surprised."

I sat quietly for a moment. *Moved.* "This is amazing. We have just heard from all six healers about patients who are cancer free, beyond all usual expectations. And more connected to their life force. What wonderful work this is."

Basking in the afterglow of these amazing patient stories, it was clear that we were part of something greater. A wave of peace ran through me. *This is indeed the final piece to fall into place—we are ready to share our experience.*

We had successfully helped our patients forge a spiritual healing connection and they were living healthier and more fulfilling lives than ever before. The next step was to document and package our approach and experience in a format that other health care providers would be able to implement.

I assembled our team and we began the work of designing materials that communicated the components of our Healing-Space program for Survivorship and how it could be implemented by other health care providers and their patients. As we moved into this project, stories began to reach us of patients who had discovered a healing connection when faced with a cancer diagnosis, outside of whatever medical care they were receiving, or in some cases when they refused medical care, or were refused further treatment. I was dismayed by the way in which the healing connection and medicine were so completely separate from one another. From the patient's perspective, it often seemed that medicine was somehow blind and deaf to the impact of their healing efforts. *How could we bridge the gap?*

As soon as I posed this question, I began to have more opportunities to talk with doctors. Dr. Schink arranged several meetings with doctors, researchers, and administrators at Northwestern where I could share our experience. I presented our cases of cancer that recovered beyond the usual expectation, and the response was powerful. They began to consider how this might be integrated into their medical setting.

Soon thereafter I attended a conference at the University of Chicago (where I completed my OB/GYN residency) and had an opportunity to talk about our work with the doctors there. It became apparent to me that there was not as much of a gap as I had first perceived. Doctors were open to the ideas I was sharing; I just needed to give them a framework for incorporating them into their thinking. Because I was a doctor who still practiced medicine, health care professionals were open to my inclusive conception.

Doctors actually rely on the healing connection, but it isn't generally part of their awareness. When surgeons operate, they take it for granted that healing will ensue. They do their thing and the body takes over. This is true for any treatment. Doctors assume that the body will respond with healing. When patients recover exceptionally well, or have unforeseen negative results, doctors don't have an explanation. Medical training is focused on specific actions steps for each diagnosis.

I found that giving doctors a model for practicing medicine while incorporating energy healing intrigued them. I began to trust myself to share with them in a way they could embrace, and I began to hear, "We could use your methods in our institution."

Currently, these talks are ongoing, but implementing the new practices is still a challenge. Healthcare delivery systems are entrenched, and introducing a new program is an enormous change. It requires a paradigm shift.

I continue to have opportunities to talk to doctors—on airplanes, at parties, wherever I am.

Recently, my daughter Olivia was seriously ill and had to be hospitalized just as we arrived out east for her senior year of college. We connected with a Hematology/Oncology physician who was helpful and supportive in her recovery. As we were closing a rather long conversation about my daughter's condition, he said, "I Googled you, and I am so impressed with your work. Would you consider coming back to Massachusetts sometime to talk to our oncology group about what you are doing?"

Here was another confirmation that I was opening a bridge between these separate worlds.

"I would love to," I said.

"Every cell in your body has a direct relationship with Creative Life Force, and each cell is independently responding. When you feel joy, all the circuits are open and the Life Force or God Force can be fully received. When you feel guilt or blame or fear or anger, the circuits are hindered and the Life Force cannot flow as effectively. Physical experience is about monitoring those circuits and keeping them as open as possible. The cells know what to do. They are summoning the Energy."

— Esther Hicks

About the Author

OVER THE LAST 38 years Marilyn Mitchell, M.D. has grown a unique medical practice that integrates Energy Healing and holistic practices with traditional medicine. She is an expert in women's health and integrative medicine, and has treated over 30,000 women and men in the Chicagoland area who are thriving with this approach. Dr. Mitchell is an intuitive, educator, speaker and health visionary. She has been a leader in the field of integrative medicine and a passionate advocate for the importance of combining energy healing with holistic and traditional medical care, partnering with the medical community to establish guiding principles for the future of healthcare. Currently she is developing on-line educational programs for healers and medical practitioners to increase their intuitive and healing abilities when dealing with seriously ill patients, and offering programs for anyone who wants to access their inner vital energy for true healing.

Connect with Marilyn Mitchell
MD/Healer

www.MarilynMitchellMD.com

Speaker
Healers: train to work in medical settings
Medical Practitioners: learn about intuitive healing
Courses and workshops

Inquire about healing
www.HealingSpaceLLC.com
info@HealingSpaceLLC.com

847-304-5526

CPSIA information can be obtained
at www.ICGtesting.com
Printed in the USA
FSHW011947120419